Shawn —

MW01281945

EAT
THAT MONKEY

Reading Eat That Monkey
can + will change your
life. Live the life you
desire... make it great!

Glen D. Porter

EAT

THAT MONKEY

Now Is the Time to Change Your Life!

Erica D. Porter
Lifestyle & Weight Management Coach, Personal Trainer,
Professional Wrestler

iUniverse, Inc.
New York Lincoln Shanghai

Eat That Monkey
Now Is the Time to Change Your Life!

iUniverse books may be ordered through booksellers or by contacting:

iUniverse
2021 Pine Lake Road, Suite 100
Lincoln, NE 68512
www.iuniverse.com
1-800-Authors (1-800-288-4677)

The information, ideas, and suggestions in this book are not intended as a substitute for professional medical advice. Before following any suggestions contained in this book, you should consult your personal physician. Neither the author nor the publisher shall be liable or responsible for any loss or damage allegedly arising as a consequence of your use or application of any information or suggestions in this book.

The views expressed in this work are solely those of the author and do not necessarily reflect the views of the publisher, and the publisher hereby disclaims any responsibility for them.

ISBN: 978-0-595-41851-0 (pbk)
ISBN: 978-0-595-86196-5 (ebk)

Printed in the United States of America

Caution:
If you are looking to drop 20 pounds in two weeks, this book is not for you. This book is for those who wish to make long lasting changes.

Acknowledgements

Thank you to the believers.

MOMD, you know who you are, thank you for being the best friend I could ever have; I love you with all that I am and more.

Dad, now that you could recite the book verbatim, after taking the time to review the book and make invaluable suggestions, it's finally done … I'll let you know when you can retire. You have always been my biggest supporter and I have the utmost respect for you. Additionally, if anyone needs an amazing photographer contact my father Wayne Porter at www.maryland-real-estate.com.

Mom, your skepticism created the drive to ensure I wrote the best book possible. I love you and I know you always want the best for me. When I am in my sixties, I want to be as beautiful, sexy, and fit as my Mother.

I cannot forget the wonderful artist who put up with all my crazy concepts and created the cover that I wanted and love … thank you Fancy Pants Francie!

Phil Huey, thank you for your friendship and putting together a magnificent website www.EatThatMonkey.com. If anyone needs an excellent website builder, Phil's your Man, phhhl@yahoo.com. He is also the founder and creator of www.junglegrrrl.net.

Where would I be if it weren't for my clients? I would like to extend a special thank you to all of you who have trusted me to assist you on a life changing journey and for being the catalysts of this project. Each of you contributed in some way whether you know it or not.

To all my friends and family, I love you! I couldn't imagine living my life without you. My parents encouraged me to be what I wanted, and hey … I'm doing it! Dreams do come true, if you want them badly enough! Thank you.

Contents

PART 1

Positive Thinking and Monkey Business

Chapter One

What Is <u>Your</u> Monkey?

"The way you live your life, the perspective you select, is a choice you make every single day when you wake up. It's yours to decide."
~Lance Armstrong

"No man is free who is not master of himself."
~Epictetus (Greek philosopher, c. 100 C.E.)

"Desire is the key to motivation, but it's the determination and commitment to an unrelenting pursuit of your goal, a commitment to excellence, that will enable you to attain the success you seek."
~Mario Andretti

You may be asking yourself, what is the "monkey" to which this woman refers? I'm glad you asked. Many people have a monkey on their back that weighs them down, figuratively and sometimes literally. Often that monkey manifests itself as added pounds blamed on a lack of knowledge or willpower, low self-esteem, laziness, self-doubt, or depression—but the monkey is there, and usually it is a combination of things. Many times our monkey intensifies because of weight gain. Because of depression, we eat to comfort ourselves, and then we pack on the weight, which sends our depression spiraling out of control.

Perhaps you are one of those people who will empty a box of cookies and immediately feel guilt, shame, and self-hatred, but repeat this behavior over and over. I wrote this book to help you gain the courage and the discipline to get that monkey off your back and change your life, both physically and mentally. I want to inspire and encourage you to embrace a life of total wellness through awareness, acceptance, and knowledge. *Now* is the time to change your life.

This book will not put you on a specific eating plan for two weeks or give you a list of fat-burning foods. However, this book will empower you to take control of your eating and exercise habits. You have the ability to control these areas of your life if you choose to do so. Trying is not enough. The only way to accomplish something is to do it, by doing whatever it takes, to keep making the effort until you reach your goal. Stop trying and start taking whatever action is necessary to reach your goal. This is effective and more than possible in *every* area of your life. Assess where you are, where you want to be, and therefore what you will need to do to get to where you want to be.

Over the next couple of chapters, I am going to help you identify your monkey and help you rid yourself of him (now men, this is not a sexist comment; I simply call every animal *him*, just as I call every car *she*). You have to look deep within yourself to identify and then take the necessary action to rid yourself of your monkey. You have to take responsibility for yourself and your actions. Getting that monkey off your back is a life-long journey that you have to work at and support every day to ensure that he does not become a permanent fixture. Each person needs a goal that is worthy of himself or herself. Living an unhealthy life takes just as much effort as living a healthy one. Anything worth having, or doing, or being, requires some effort on your part.

We have much more control over our lives than we want to accept; moreover, what we put in our mouth is completely under our control! You have no excuse. You have the choice whether to eat grilled or baked instead of fried, fruit instead of cheesecake, flavored water instead of soda, skim milk instead of full fat milk—choices no one can deny you. Do not allow your food to control you; take control of your food! Be aware of your behaviors, for example, shoveling food in your mouth without thought. Unfortunately, mindless eating translates to added weight on the scale. Your top priority must be yourself and your health; after all, you get only one body, so treat it like a temple, a diamond in the rough. You cannot get the body you want if you don't respect the body you have. Explore why you have not been successful in the past. Love your body and its capabilities. Focus on living the healthiest life, not being the thinnest. Live the life you deserve. Each day you have choices to make—choices that will dictate your actions. You choose whether you want to make a change. You choose whether you want to be in control. You choose whether you want to speak positively about yourself.

Why do I feel it is crucial for you to address your monkey and start living a healthy life? Diabetes[1], hypertension (or high blood pressure)[2], heart disease[3], and so many other killer problems are at all-time highs because people are not taking responsibility for their health. Do the thoughts of blindness, dialysis, amputation, stroke, heart attack, or debilitating arthritis mean anything to you? These are serious complications associated with the above diseases that can increase with your weight; don't allow them to affect *your* life. In many cases, if you suffer from any of these symptoms you may still have the power to change a

1. Julie Louise Gerberding, MD, MPH, "At a Glance 2006: Diabetes: Disabling, Deadly, and on the Rise," Centers for Disease Control and Prevention, available online, http://www.cdc.gov/nccdphp/publications/aag/ddt.htm, December 6, 2006.

2. American Heart Association, http://www.americanheart.org/, July 13, 2006.

3. American Heart Association, http://www.americanheart.org/, July 13, 2006.

devastating outcome. Now is the time to make the necessary changes in order to live your healthiest life. It's not too late to get your health back on track—**it's not too late**. Make the choice to improve your health through better nutrition and/or exercise (increased movement)! Get that monkey off your back.

As with most aspects of our lives, our eating and exercise habits develop at an early age. Some of these habits are good, and some we should change. Fortunately, the human brain can be retrained and redirected, so you can modify destructive behaviors through action, patience, experimentation, and commitment. One of the reasons most fad diets on the market are so horrible is that they do not allow you to deviate from their menu and find what is *right* for *you*. Neither do they offer any real long-term help. You will need to make lifestyle changes that take time—you can achieve this by addressing and removing your monkey and empowering yourself. You will realize that being in control of what you put into your body will produce physiological and psychological benefits that make you feel stronger, more attractive, more energized, and healthier, and they will give you an overwhelming sense of accomplishment.

Become educated on nutrition and exercise and change your life. However, it is a lifelong commitment, not a two-week gimmick. There are countless resources at your disposal to help you become educated, including the Internet and the library. I highly recommend the *Nutrition Action Healthletter*, and you can find out more about it by visiting the link www.cspinet.org. Some other helpful links are www.health. harvard.edu/Wellness_and_Prevention/, www.naturalhealthmag.com, and www.prevention.com. *Nothing* will keep you from achieving success when you have the proper knowledge and most importantly—the desire.

What makes my approach better than that of Atkins, Agatsons (author of *The South Beach Diet*), and all the others who claim to hold the "key" to weight loss? This: I am not looking to generate millions of dollars with a one-size-fits-all diet. I want to help you become well informed and make the choices that will improve your life for the long haul. I will give you the information and the tools necessary to achieve lifelong success. You will accomplish this by learning to make changes for today, tomorrow, and then the rest of your life. This is not a temporary quick fix.

The diet books that fill the bookstore shelves are the reason you are reading my book now. They always wind up failing and letting you down. Willpower is not the only issue; you must be practical when making any lifestyle change, especially in your eating and exercise habits. Come on, be honest with yourself—can you eliminate carbohydrates for the rest of your life? I certainly cannot. No *one* food makes you fat; *fat is the result of too much food! As a result of modern conveniences, we are moving less and burning fewer calories.* I am not recreating the wheel. Science and common sense support these facts.

So, I want you to *think and reflect—what is your monkey?* Are you someone who overeats? Someone who does not exercise? Someone who loves sweets and has no self-control around them? Someone who eats out of boredom? Someone who eats too fast? Someone who associates food with pleasant experiences? Someone who simply does not understand how to eat? Someone who was taught to clean your plate? Someone who eats with distractions like the TV? What is *your* monkey? *The first step toward getting that monkey off your back is to acknowledge your monkey and commit to learning healthful habits.* Start visualizing the life you want for yourself. While I encourage you to get down to your healthy weight, you must manage separating the number on the scale from your self-worth. Now, join me on this journey of self-realization and self-awareness!

Table 1:

<u>Behavior Modification:</u> (Choose **One** behavior to change)
Allow as much time as needed for a change to become habit. Do not rush this process. You cannot be dependent on others to keep motivated to change, believe in yourself. Set goals that you can live with—*lifestyle* is just that, a style of life.

1. What ONE behavior do you wish to change?

2. How do you feel when you allow your behavior to control you?

3. What is the origin (root cause) of this behavior?

4. What triggers this behavior?

5. What are the benefits of changing this behavior?

6. What are the benefits of *not* changing this behavior?

7. Have you tried to change this behavior before?

8. If yes, for how long did you make the change and why did you revert to old-habits?

9. What goal(s) do you wish to accomplish by making this change?

   a. Short Term?

   b. Long Term?

10. Write Yes or No.

    a. Changing this behavior is important to *me*.

    b. I am willing to do whatever it takes to achieve this goal.

    c. I believe I will succeed in making this change.

    d. My health will be better because of making this change.

    e. I have chosen a goal that I can be successful in achieving.

    f. I am truly committed.

    g. I will ask for support.

★ You can be successful only if you wrote "yes" to all the above statements. If you wrote "no" to any of the above, I suggest you choose another behavior that will allow you to reply "yes" to all. You will have the opportunity to change all behaviors; however, you will only make one change at a time.

11. What steps will you need to take in order to succeed?

12. What obstacles might you encounter?

13. How can you overcome these obstacles?

14. What outside forces will you need to address in order to reach your goal?

15. Keep a journal and write down anything and everything related to your goal—how did you feel, what obstacles did you encounter, and how did you overcome theses obstacles, etc.

16. Post this exercise where you have to look at it every day. Use positive self-talk every time you look at your written commitment to change.

17. When you have been completely successful in changing your behavior, you will choose another behavior and repeat.

Have fun! Remember to reward yourself for achieving success (if your behavior has to do with food, I would suggest you treat yourself to something non-food related such as a massage, sports tickets, new shoes, a new golf club, or a new exercise outfit.)

Table 2 (Using Table 1):
Behavior Modification *Example.* Completed by Erica Porter.

1. What ONE behavior do you wish to change?
   My mindless overeating

2. How do you feel when you allow your behavior to control you?
   I have this feeling of self-loathing and resentment, anger, and helplessness

3. What is the origin of this behavior?
   Social acceptance

4. What triggers this behavior?
   Boredom, distractions, variety, and food accessibility

5. What are the benefits of changing this behavior?
   Weight loss, sense of control, sense of accomplishment, not feeling angry and depressed afterward

6. What are the benefits of not changing this behavior?
   I can't fail if I don't try ... nothing really

7. Have you tried to change this behavior before?
   Yes

8. If yes, how long did you make the change for and why did you revert to old-habits?

   I have tried many times and have failed because I have tried to change too many things at once and I probably didn't truly believe I could change

9. What goal(s) do you wish to accomplish by making this change?
   a. Short Term?
      Daily self-control, awareness of the experience of eating
   b. Long Term?
      Weight loss, self-control

10. Write Yes or No.
    a. Changing this behavior is important to *me. yes*
    b. I am willing to do whatever it takes to achieve this goal. *yes*
    c. I believe I will succeed in making this change. *yes*
    d. My health will be better because of making this change. *yes*
    e. I have chosen a goal that I can be successful in achieving. *yes*
    f. I am truly committed. *yes*
    g. I will ask for support. *yes*

★ You can only be successful if you wrote "yes" to all the above statements. If you wrote "no" to any of the above, I suggest you choose another behavior that will allow you to reply "yes" to all. You will have the opportunity to change all behaviors; however, you will only make one change at a time.

11. What steps will you need to take in order to succeed?

—*Keep a journal to track my emotions to determine what triggers my overeating. How am I feeling when I get the urge to splurge. Where am I? Who is with me? What are my thoughts? Am I hungry or emotional?*

—*Eat sitting at the table without distractions*

—*Serve my food on a smaller plate and put food away prior to sitting down*

—*Eat slowly and enjoy each bite*

—*Eat with chopsticks*

—*Keep healthy snacks readily available (cut veggies, apples, peeled oranges, homemade light soups)*

—*Do not nibble on the foods I am cooking*

—*Slow Down*

12. What obstacles might you encounter?

—*Parties with finger foods and buffets*

—*Working out of the house—I get bored and eat*

—*Didn't have time to eat all day and now I'm starving and will eat everything in sight*

—*Eating in a hurry for lack of time*

13. How can you overcome these obstacles?

—*Eat something healthy prior to going out, chew gum—you can't chew gum and eat*

—*Don't keep unhealthy snack foods in the house, cut up veggies, apples, oranges, and like foods to grab when I want to eat something or go for a walk if I get cravings*

—*Keep healthful snacks with me all the time to avoid overeating later*

—*Prepare healthy meals ahead of time, make a big pot of oatmeal on Sunday, so all I have to do is reheat to save time, make salads that I can take for lunch, make dishes that I can put in Tupperware containers or that can be frozen and reheated quickly*

14. What outside forces will you need to address in order to reach your goal?

    —*Telling my friends and family about my goals so that they can support me in this change*

15. Keep a journal and write down anything and everything related to your goal—how did you feel, what obstacles did you encounter and how did you overcome them, etc.

16. Post this exercise where you have to look at it every day. Use positive self-talk every time you look at your written commitment to change.

17. When you have been completely successful in changing your behavior, you will choose another behavior and repeat.

★★What do you believe to be your monkey? The behavior you would like to change or the behaviors origin (root cause)?

Eat that monkey!

Chapter Two

About Me

"Whatever your passion is in life, you set your goals and you stick to it."
~Stacy Dragila

"Don't wait for flowers to be brought to you, plant your own garden."
~Author Unknown

"I believe that we learn by practice. Whether it means to learn to dance by practicing dancing or to learn to live by practicing living, the principles are the same. In each, it is the performance of a dedicated precise set of acts, physical or intellectual, from which comes shape of achievement, a sense of one's being, a satisfaction of spirit.... Practice means to perform, over and over again in the face of all obstacles, some act of vision, of faith, of desire. Practice is a means of inviting the perfection desired."
~Martha Graham

I think it is important for you to understand who I am and why I felt it necessary to write this book. My name is Erica Porter, and I am extremely passionate about health and nutrition. I am dedicated to educating others so they can lead healthy, productive lives. I am devoted to my mission, and I never plan to stop. My motivation is motivating others to live the happiest, most fulfilling lives possible.

I enjoy food—all kinds of food. I love having dessert after dinner or occasionally eating french fries, but I get it! I know that to afford myself the things I love, I cannot go overboard—I must be in control. I have to exercise to accommodate the excess calories and while I, like most people, would love to eat cookies, ice cream, french fries, or pizza at every meal, I would weigh 500 pounds if I did not manage what I eat. Eating with enjoyment is a matter of balance and moderation. I am on this planet to enjoy myself, and therefore, I would never exclude the foods that add to that pleasure; however, I have learned to keep a healthy balance between nutritious (foods that contain vitamins, minerals, fiber, and/or protein that add to a balanced diet) and empty foods (foods that simply provide calories and add no nutritional value). While I eat the things I enjoy, I also work out. Exercise is an important part of my life, and it makes me feel strong and sexy. I like feeling healthy and good about myself.

There is an ignorance regarding basic health in our country, evidenced in the fact that I see people making horrible choices for themselves on a daily basis. Choices that affect their health and could therefore impact the lives of those around them. Is it that people do not care or that they do not want to be bothered? I ponder this because I see people at the grocery store, restaurant, or similar places making all the wrong food choices. This unawareness does not always manifest itself in weight alone. You do not have to be overweight to be unhealthy. There are plenty of "skinny fat people," as I call them, who are thin, but their health is poor because of poor diet and a lack of exercise. Poor health is a growing problem, and often if you are uneducated on the basic components of health and nutrition, chances are your parents did not have a clue, and your children will not either. You must make the effort to break the cycle of this easily reversible problem. One person can change the lives of future generations. That one person could be you.

I was fortunate that at a very young age I learned the importance of healthy eating. Both my father and mother cooked, and we sat down together to eat our meals. It was not often that we ate out, but when we did, we did not eat at McDonald's, Carl's Junior, Wendy's, Burger King, or any other food establishment of this sort; we ate a variety of different, authentic ethnic foods prepared fresh, not loaded down with preservatives and fillers. I'm glad that my parents did not take the easy road with frozen dinners and fast food. Both my parents worked, and they worked hard, but they always made time to cook and sit down and eat with us. Remember, it only takes one person to change a cycle of an unhealthy lifestyle. It has nothing to do with growing up poor or privileged; it has to do with a healthy appreciation for food and making a healthful mealtime a priority, period! It *is* possible to eat wholesomely on a fixed income. There are plenty of inexpensive ways in which to eat better.

Growing up, I was always very active. In fact, my parents did not allow us to watch much TV at all. They allowed my brother and me only thirty minutes of television viewing a night. Instead of sitting around the house, my parents encouraged us to be involved in athletics, read, and be creative (build forts, make crafts, create a play). I was extremely involved in gymnastics, swimming, and dancing, about which I became very passionate.

My enthusiasm for dance would mold me into the person I am today. During high school, I became an apprentice and then a teacher at the Backstage Dance Studio in Columbia, Maryland. I also cofounded and performed in my high school's dance squad, which still exists to this day. My experiences unquestionably drove me to want to become a professional dancer.

I went off to college to study dance, as well as biology and business management. I quickly learned the harsh realities of the dancer stereotype—some of the dance teachers at my university told me I was too fat to be a dancer. Too fat? I was a tremendous athlete, but sadly, I did not fit the mold. Being healthy was a choice, not a sacrifice, so I refused to give into the self-destruction and eating disorders that took hold of many of my peers in the dance world. What a sad thing to have to let go of your dreams because the industry cannot manage talent versus body type properly. During this time, I became increasingly aware and intrigued with the human body, so I became a certified personal trainer, which launched my quest to improve people's health.

During my four years in college, I learned that my integrity was everything. I was in command of myself, and the person I would become. I learned the true meaning of self-confidence and self-respect. After I received my Bachelor of Arts, I headed to Los Angeles to work in dance. Unfortunately, the dancer's stereotype was not just prevalent in Pittsburgh—it was everywhere. I was not going to let this destroy me; I simply had to figure out what I was going to do with my life now that I was three thousand miles from the place I had called home.

I dabbled in many different things to find my calling. I worked for a health club as a trainer and a sales consultant. Helping people take control and recognize a positive change in their lives is what motivates me.

After the gym, I began training clients on my own and continued my search for other inspirational careers. I went back to my roots of teaching kids dance and gymnastics. Rather than be stuck at one location, I would pack my little car full of mats, hula-hoops, beanbags, and such things, and travel from school to school. Not easy work, but extremely rewarding. I will always remain active in helping to shape the lives of children through movement and positive influence.

About two years later, a friend informed me of an audition for athletic women, and of course, I was intrigued enough to go. Turns out it was for an all-women's wrestling show, and since you do not know my personality, you will have to trust me when I say that this was a perfect fit. This opportunity allowed me to combine all the things I loved: performing, athleticism, and being the center of attention. I had found my calling at last. I know, most people are thinking—professional wrestler? Yes, professional wrestler. Wrestling demands top-notch athleticism and total dedication because you are putting the lives of yourself and your co-workers at risk. It is entertainment, but fake it is not, and there are risks. This was a once-in-a-lifetime opportunity, and I took full advantage.

During this time, I landed a role in the first Spiderman movie as a Bonnette in the wrestling scene. The scene occurs right after Spiderman has the "with great power comes great responsibility" talk with his uncle. I am the last girl to yell at Spidey, and I hand Macho Man Randy Savage the chair he uses to hit Spiderman. You can visit www.junglegrrrl.net for an inside look. The wrestling industry helped me to make some great contacts that have allowed me to continue working in the field of sports entertainment. Most recently, I have been involved with motion capturing for wrestling video games. In addition, I do regular work with various programs on *The Learning Channel*, *The Travel Channel*, and *Fox Sports Net*.

I also continue teaching dance to both children and adults. During the 2005 Women's National Basketball Association season, I worked with *The Los Angeles SparKids* (a group of dancers ages twelve to eighteen that perform during time-outs and halftime at the Los Angeles Sparks home games) as the assistant to the director.

Being involved in such a physical line of work keeps me aware of my body and health. It has also made me extremely sensitive to the distorted and self-deprecating influence that the entertainment business has on people in and out of its circle. The exposure to all aspects of "body obsession" has been extremely interesting.

I have been traveling abroad to countries such as Colombia, Ecuador, Germany, Italy, Netherlands, and South Korea since I was young, and I have seen firsthand the societal differences regarding eating. When I am visiting other countries, the absentmindedness of the people in my own country becomes more apparent. People in other countries eat to live, not live to eat. They take more time to enjoy their meals, eat whole foods, and even eat cheese and bread and drink wine. If I recall correctly, many of the popular diet books state that bread is evil and makes people fat. There is not one food that makes people fat—too much of anything makes people fat. Lack of movement makes people fat. You do not need to eat salad at every meal or run a marathon to reap the benefits of a healthier lifestyle. Each person has different nutritional needs and requirements. If you feel you are suffering from an illness that makes losing weight more difficult please consult with a physician. I understand that some people have specific medical conditions that make losing weight more difficult, but many people throw in the towel and admit defeat because they think optimal health is impossible for them—not true. You did not invite your monkey, yet you allow him to stay!

You might ask, what is Erica Porter's monkey? Yes, I too have a monkey. I have battled excessive overeating for most of my teenage and adult years. I have a love/hate relationship with food. My friends were always amazed at how much food I could consume without gaining weight, but I would take it too far. Because people found my food consumption so intriguing (and I liked the attention), I would go overboard and eventually began to lose control of my eating habits. My monkey had arrived. I have gone through the self-loathing and depression associated with feeling out of control. I do not like this feeling. I am a person that needs a lot, if not total, control. I am aware of this through self-analysis, and I have to work at it every day, otherwise it is very easy to slip back into old habits, which I know would be doing myself a disservice if I allowed that to happen. So you see, my monkey is social acceptance and needing attention. Do you have a similar story?

Through all my endeavors, current and past, I have learned that what makes me happiest is educating people on becoming healthy and helping them understand how to rid themselves of their monkey. I remain committed to learning and understanding health and nutrition, and I have continued my education by becoming a Lifestyle and Weight Management Specialist. My work helps me remain grounded and true to myself. I do not know everything and do not pretend to, but I make it a point to learn something new everyday and listen to people's needs and desires. Every person I have worked with has a different need, a different desire, and a different goal; they each have their monkey to remove. It gives me great pleasure to "tag team" that monkey with them! If you expect the best from yourself, then you are more likely to get it. Now, I want to help you be your best!

Chapter Three

Positive Is the Key. No *Body* Is Perfect

"Hold up your head! You were not made for failure, you were made for victory. Go forward with a joyful confidence"
~George Eliot

"There is no pleasure in life equal to that of the conquest of a vicious habit."
~Author Unknown

"… If there is something out there that you want to do … don't focus on the obstacles. Don't ask for permission. Just dive in."
~John Wood

Cosmetic surgeries, weight loss surgeries, diet pills, and diet book sales are skyrocketing, and for what—to strive for perfection with as little effort as possible? For whose definition of beauty are we striving? The "perfect" person does not exist, and what each person finds beautiful is different—at least, you hope it would be. Have we become a society that only allows for one type of beauty? As cliché as it sounds, you can only find happiness and beauty in other people when you are happy with yourself. Of course, you can only find happiness and beauty in yourself once you love and accept yourself. This, of course, is the tricky part. What is happiness for you? If you are unhappy with something, change it. If you are out of control, help yourself get in control. A healthy body is going to begin with a healthy attitude. However, many people fail to address their underlying issue(s)—their monkey—and opt instead for superficial changes. The change has to come from within first if you ever desire real change on the outside. Weight loss will not change the person you want to be, but addressing your monkey will help you achieve the health you deserve.

For many, the biggest obstacle to true happiness is their weight. Luckily, your weight is within your control, but you must accept this responsibility, because if you don't the sad, ugly cycle of dieting creates self-loathing, which inescapably makes your monkey heavier. The idea that you have to be slim and fit—whatever it takes—is upsetting and counterproductive; a healthy lifestyle will not come in the form of a magic pill or fast-acting diet book. Wake up, people! The diet industry is making a magic million while you fail again. There is *no* magic pill, only consistent effort and dedication! You must eat your monkey!

Envision putting on a big backpack. Each time you doubt yourself, call yourself a name, allow someone else's hurtful words to affect you, or say, "I can't," you put a brick in the bag. This bag gets awfully heavy for most people. This is what we are doing to ourselves: we are letting that monkey get heavier and heavier. Nevertheless, you can get rid of that monkey, because *you* have the choice. You will feel liberated and light. Learn to take care of yourself emotionally—step-by-step and day-by-day—and eventually you will rid yourself of your monkey and be the happy, healthy person you have always dreamed you could be.

Are you one of the "big, beautiful, and proud?" Perhaps this is how you truly feel or perhaps you have accepted this motto because you have attempted to lose weight and have "failed." Either way, your health is most important and you should take responsibility to change your health for the better. I am certainly not saying you have to be 5' 10" and weigh 115 pounds; however, if you are 5' 2" and weigh 200 pounds, you are overweight! I have tremendous respect for someone who has great self-confidence, but if you are overweight, you are prone to increasing health problems, and I cannot imagine that you are truly happy with the way that you *feel*. This is not about the way one looks, but rather about one's health. Think about the risks associated with being overweight. Do you want to lead a healthy life, or an unhealthy one? Man or woman, healthy is good—not perfection—healthy! You must focus on how your body feels, not how it looks. When you focus on making your body feel better, looking better will usually be a natural result.

Some things will be difficult to change. For example, some women and even some men have cellulite, but there are ways to look better that I have addressed in the exercise portion of this book. You can reshape the body, if you want. Again, this is a matter of choice—what do you choose?

In order to achieve true happiness and optimal health, we must quit looking at magazines and getting depressed because we do not look like the "models" filling the pages. You know what? Most of those people do not look like those people (check out Dove's Real Beauty campaign: http://www.campaignforrealbeauty.ca/film_fullscreen_evo.html). First, a professional whose job is to make them look extraordinary makes up the models in the magazines. Then there are people who create the perfect lighting to capture the most desirable images. When the makeup and lighting do not hide all the flaws, specialists retouch the photos, so that you and I end up feeling like crap. Great—now that you understand how it works, do not torture yourself by comparing. When you have the money to employ these professionals to do a photo shoot for you, you will realize how magnificent you can look as well.

Realize the people in the magazines, on television, and in the movies make sacrifices to look the way they do, usually unhealthy and sometimes dangerous ones. There is a model named Carrie Otis who made her story and struggle public. She spoke of the crash diets and cocaine she used to look picture perfect. She became addicted to heroin. She would hardly eat anything two weeks prior to a photo shoot, and she would run seven miles a day. Clearly, her lifestyle was unsustainable, and therefore she needed to get her monkey off her back. She has had to fight to create a lifestyle that supports her happiness and incorporate many of the concepts I share with you in this book. While her situation may be an extreme example compared with yours, the only real difference is the speed and intensity with which she reached a dead-end. If you do not make changes, you too may find yourself at a dead-end.

There are plenty of celebrities that are now sharing their stories as well: Delta Burke, Elton John, Mariel Hemingway, Oprah Winfrey, Paula Abdul, the late Princess Diana, Ruben Studdard, Tracy Gold, and Wynonna Judd—just to name a few. Oprah Winfrey continues to struggle with disordered eating. Oprah said about her weight, "It's always a struggle. I've felt safer and more protected when I was heavy. Food has always been comforting."[1] Diana, Princess of Wales, struggled with an eating disorder. The following is from an interview that Princess Diana gave about her battle with bulimia—"I had bulimia for a number of years. And that's like a secret disease. You inflict it upon yourself because your self-esteem is at a low ebb, and you don't think you're worthy or valuable. You fill your stomach up four or five times a day—some do it more—and it gives you a feeling of comfort. It's like having a pair of arms around you, but it's temporarily, temporary. Then you're disgusted at the bloatedness of your stomach, and then you bring it all up again. And it's a repetitive pattern, which is very destructive to yourself."[2] Country singer Wynonna Judd struggles with emotional eating and is

1.   EDReferral.com (eating disorder referral.com), "Famous celebrities who have spoken publicly about their suffering with Eating Disorders," December 1, 2006.

2.   Princess of Wales, Interview by Martin Bashir, BBC News, available online http://www.bbc.co.uk/politics97/diana/panorama.html, September 14, 2006.

on her journey toward healthy eating. "It's not about size, I'll let that take care of itself. The work I'm doing is inside. The physical will follow the mental and spiritual and emotional." In her book *Coming Home to Myself*, Wynonna tells her story and gives readers an honest insight into her life and emotions.[3] So as you see, no one is immune to falling victim to his or her monkey.

We have a tendency to look up to celebrities and wish for what they have. I certainly do not want these people's lives or struggles. Make changes for yourself and not because of what you see in a picture of someone else that is not, and will never be, you. *You* are *beautiful.* I, for one, am happy that I do not have to live my life as a perfect model; however, I continuously do my best to be happy with myself, first as a whole, and then the naked woman I see in the mirror. I am beautiful but not perfect. I have some fat on my gluteus maximus, and my tummy has a little puff to it. I certainly do not look anything like the women in magazines, but I look good. I am healthy because I eat well most of the time, and I exercise on a regular basis. I am able to enjoy myself because I can breathe easily, sit in a regular size seat comfortably, and engage in almost any activity. When I walk down the street, people notice me for all the right reasons—because I hold my head up high and know that I am true to myself and in control. My best is always under construction. Most importantly, I live my life the way I encourage others to live theirs.

Being thin is not the answer to all your problems. In fact, I know many thin women who are extremely unhappy and unhealthy. So, make the effort to improve your health. Trust me when I say you will be happier if you work on your *whole* self, especially if your weight issue is due to unhappiness, mindless eating, and binges. So, please, get out of the habit of comparing yourself with other people. You have control over yourself, and that is all that should matter.

Most people have a tendency to compare themselves with others or put others down when they are not feeling good about their *self.* Does

---

3.   "Celebrities and the media, the pressure to be thin," http://www.eating-disorder-information.com/mediacelebrities.asp, November 20, 2006, accessed on February 19, 2007.

this ever actually make you feel better? There will always be someone who is more attractive, thinner, or smarter, but confident people will embrace these qualities in others, not discourage them. Confident people tend to praise others and do not react to negativity. Confidence has nothing to do with being the most beautiful, the thinnest, the most talented, or the smartest; it has everything to do with accepting and loving everything there is to you. *Learn to love and accept the whole you—your strengths and your weaknesses.*

Table 3 Written Exercise:

<u>Learn to love and accept the whole you—your strengths and your weaknesses</u>

1. Select: (I am _____ in this area.)

1-<u>Excellent</u> 2-<u>Good, but could use work</u> 3-<u>Desperately in need of help</u>

___Accepting	___Flexible
___Ambitious (Motivated)	___Forgiving
___Aspiring	___Goal Oriented
___Believing in myself	___Mature
___Believing in others	___Objective
___Change (I accept and embrace change)	___Open-Minded
___Cheerful	___Patient
___Conscious of Weaknesses	___Reliable
___Considerate of others	___Self-Confident
___Considerate of myself	___Self-Disciplined
___Decisive	___Self-Esteem
___Enthusiastic	___Self-Reliant

2. Now, write the traits as you numbered them in the appropriately numbered columns:

	<u>1</u>	<u>2</u>	<u>3</u>
1.			
2.			
3.			
4.			
5.			
6.			
7.			
8.			
9.			
10.			
11.			
12.			
13.			
14.			
15.			
16.			
17.			
18.			
19.			
20.			
21.			
22.			
23.			
24.			
25.			

Choose *one* trait that is most desperately in need of help. You will now use the *Behavior Modification* (Table 1) exercise from Chapter 1 (see below) to complete the remainder of this exercise. *Your trait is the behavior you wish to change.

Table 1:

Behavior Modification: (Choose **One** behavior to change)
Allow as much time as needed for a change to become habit. Do not rush this process. You cannot be dependent on others to keep motivated to change, believe in yourself. Set goals that you can live with—*lifestyle* is just that, a style of life.

1. What ONE behavior do you wish to change?
2. How do you feel when you allow your behavior to control you?
3. What is the origin (root cause) of this behavior?
4. What triggers this behavior?
5. What are the benefits of changing this behavior?
6. What are the benefits of *not* changing this behavior?
7. Have you tried to change this behavior before?
8. If yes, for how long did you make the change and why did you revert to old-habits?
9. What goal(s) do you wish to accomplish by making this change?
   a. Short Term?
   b. Long Term?
10. Write Yes or No.
   a. Changing this behavior is important to *me*.
   b. I am willing to do whatever it takes to achieve this goal.
   c. I believe I will succeed in making this change.
   d. My health will be better because of making this change.

e. I have chosen a goal that I can be successful in achieving.

f. I am truly committed.

g. I will ask for support.

★ You can be successful only if you wrote "yes" to all the above statements. If you wrote "no" to any of the above, I suggest you choose another behavior that will allow you to reply "yes" to all. You will have the opportunity to change all behaviors; however, you will only make one change at a time.

11. What steps will you need to take in order to succeed?

12. What obstacles might you encounter?

13. How can you overcome these obstacles?

14. What outside forces will you need to address in order to reach your goal?

15. Keep a journal and write down anything and everything related to your goal—how did you feel, what obstacles did you encounter, and how did you overcome theses obstacles, etc.

16. Post this exercise where you have to look at it every day. Use positive self-talk every time you look at your written commitment to change.

17. When you have been completely successful in changing your behavior, you will choose another behavior and repeat.

Have fun! Remember to reward yourself for achieving success (if your behavior has to do with food, I would suggest you treat yourself to something non-food related such as a massage, sports tickets, new shoes, a new golf club, or a new exercise outfit.)

Learn to change your negative thoughts into positive thoughts. An important step to self-confidence and acceptance is becoming a *can* person, because *can't* is a self-defeating thought pattern that keeps us from improving. *Can't* simply means you *won't*. There is no such thing as *can't* if you *want*. Negative people start believing what they are telling themselves: I can't eat well, I can't stop eating McDonald's, and I can't lose weight. Don't handicap your efforts with this negative self-talk! When you focus on the negative, the law of attraction says you will receive more of the same—negative. Therefore, if you want positive in your life, you must exude positivity. Change the negative behavior and tell yourself, *I can!* Your words have power in them; you will believe the things you tell yourself or how you talk about yourself to others. Choose the words "I am," and then what you want—I am beautiful, I am great, I am healthy, I am fit, and I am the best—I *am!*

There are *zero* negative consequences to eating better and moving more! *None.* What you will get is a better quality of life. No more excuses. Believe you can live a healthier life and set priorities accordingly. Tell yourself, "I *can!*" Remember, you did not simply jump up and start walking as a child. You stumbled and fell on your face and then got up and tried again. A friend of mine has a saying that she put on her *Spiritual Fitness Wear* clothing line (www.spiritualfitnesswear.com): "If you fall on your face, at least you're moving forward." You are never going to know everything, and you are bound to make mistakes, so be that child again and learn to walk. Remember my saying, "Your best is always under construction." A healthier life is a positive change, so free yourself and get that monkey off your back!

Visualize what you want for yourself. What you want can be within your grasp if you have a vision of what you want and then you take the necessary action to achieve that vision.

➤ Visualization:

"We all use imagery every day when we engage in the two most common forms of worry: either regretting the past or fearing the future …

we can use that same ability in a more positive way—for example, by imagining a tropical vacation we want to take, or a room we want to redecorate.… The more you bring your attention, or conscious awareness, to something you intend to manifest, the more likely that intention will become real in the world."

~Candace B. Pert, PhD

See Less *(C-Less)* **of yourself**
Confidence
Loving Yourself
Energy
Strength
Stamina

- When you visualize the things you want, achieving them becomes more tangible.
- What do you have to do in order to achieve the result?
- You must believe what you are visualizing and take action.
- If you wish for your health to be better, does it make sense to eat french fries and donuts on a daily basis?
- Do the words that you speak match the action you take?

★ Now that you have a vision, the *Behavioral Modification* exercise will mean even more.

Would you agree that you need to be motivated in order to change your life? Would you agree that motivation is a thought and that without action, your motivation is nothing? I learned that in order to be motivated, I must first take *action*! When I first thought about writing this book, I was consumed by negative thoughts—all the work and hours I would be putting into it with no near-term financial benefit. People even asked me about it, and I said, "Oh, I am getting to it." You know what happened: as soon as I sat down and started writing, I became highly motivated. The writing became easy and fun and I realized my hard work would be worthwhile. I took action! If you want an "A" on a test, you must study. If you want a promotion at work, you must do more than just show up to work. If you want to go on a trip, you must prepare before arriving at the airport. So, do not just think about the things you want to change or achieve; take action and make them happen.

Gain control of your *self* and your *life*. Believe in yourself and your power to change unhealthy behaviors. Get that monkey off your back. You *can*! Address your monkey and take action. It truly is as simple as it sounds. By taking action, you may require the assistance of outside forces (husband, wife, partner, doctor, or nutritionist). You must become in touch with your feelings and your desires. Respect yourself and allow for growth. Set lofty goals, achieve them, and repeat! Throw fear out the window; do not allow it to control you. Take it one day at a time, and before you know it, you will be climbing Mount Everest and feeling great! Free yourself from limitations. Believe you *can* succeed. Repeat: I will, and I can. Be free to live, free to be healthy, and free to be happy! Eat that monkey!

Chapter Four

The Fattening of America

"We are what we repeatedly do. Excellence then, is not an act, but a habit."
~Aristotle

"Great changes may not happen right away, but with effort even the difficult may become easy."
~Bill Blackman

"Courage is believing in yourself, and that is something no one can teach you."
~El Cordobes

Obesity is the second leading cause of preventable death in the United States. The estimate for excess deaths due to obesity ranges from 112,000 per year to 365,000 per year.[1] The rising rate of obesity certainly does not reflect any new genetic transformation. Rather, it is a sign of social behavior. We no longer work jobs that require physical labor; instead, we work long hours in offices, sitting at desks, which requires little or no movement. While our movement has declined, our food consumption has gone up due to excessive portions and calorie-laden foods.

Before death, come the medical visits and bills. Obesity's financial toll is steep. Over the past two decades, obesity has become a public health crisis of epidemic proportions in the United States. About one-third of U.S. adults, ages twenty and older, are overweight—68.5 million (34.1 percent). Nearly one-third of U.S. adults are obese—64.7 million (32.2 percent).[2] Overweight and obesity are associated with increased morbidity and mortality, and they exact significant economic costs. In 2000, the estimated total cost of obesity in the United States was $117 billion. About $61 billion was for direct medical costs, and $56 billion was for indirect costs.[3]

Furthermore, both the healthy and unhealthy share in the cost of insurance rates. Roland Sturm used regression analysis to show that obese adults incur annual medical expenditures that are $395 (36 percent) higher than those of normal weight incur.[4] This analysis, however, was limited to people under age sixty-five. People age sixty-five and older now account for roughly one-fourth of the obese population, and

1.   Katherine M. Flegal, PhD; Barry I. Graubard, PhD; David F. Williamson, PhD; Mitchell H. Gail, MD, PhD, "Excess Deaths Associated With Underweight, Overweight, and Obesity," *Journal of the American Medical Association,* Vol. 293 No. 15, April 20, 2005.

2.   Ogden CL, Carroll MD, Curtin LR, McDowell MA, Tabak CJ, Flegal KM. "Prevalence of overweight and obesity in the United States, 1999–2004," *Journal of the American Medical Association.* 2006; 295:1549–1555.

3.   "Preventing Obesity and Chronic Diseases Through Good Nutrition and Physical Activity," http://www.cdc.gov/nccdphp/publications/factsheets/Prevention/obesity.htm, February 21, 2006.

4.   R. Sturm, "The Effects of Obesity, Smoking, and Drinking on Medical Problems and Costs," *Health Affairs* (Mar/Apr 2002): 245–253.

because of the chronic nature of obesity-attributable diseases, medical spending for treating elderly obese people is likely to be much higher than spending for nonelderly obese people. Many of these issues are a matter of lifestyle choice—the choice is yours.

Your death certificate will not list "unhealthy lifestyle" as the cause, but chances are, if you are leading an unhealthy life, that *is* what will kill you. Obesity is a *killer*, plaguing people with debilitating ailments and boosting health care costs. There is no reason for this epidemic. It is time to work towards prevention rather than having to rely on medications for stability. We need to address our monkeys and work toward liberating ourselves from *them*. Unfortunately, most people want a magic pill to do the work for them, something that requires no effort on their part. Sadly, this trend shows no sign of slowing down. When does it stop? It stops now; it stops with you! You must eat your monkey!

My desire for you is to examine your current choices. As a nation, we are getting fatter and fatter! The Center for Disease Control and Prevention has found obesity's rate of increase to be the same in each state between both sexes regardless of age, race, or educational level.[5] *Choice* is one of the most significant differentiators among people regardless of race, sex, or age—despite the fact that particular foods figure more predominantly in certain races and communities, increasing the health risks among those people. These people still have choices. Everyone has the choice to opt for a healthier alternative in most of the foods they eat—grilled instead of fried, mustard instead of mayo, salad (with a little lemon, or oil and vinegar) instead of french fries, and to cut back on salt. In addition to one's food choices, most of us have the ability to add movement into our lives. If you live in an unsafe area, create an indoor workout for yourself. You can do push-ups, sit-ups, jog in place, climb stairs, and even curl food cans. Make the choices that have a positive impact on your health.

What about the choices we make that have a negative impact. Do you think the diet industry is helping the obesity problem or perpetuating it? A

---

5.   Eric Schlosser, Fast Food Nation: The Dark Side of the American Meal, Boston: Houghton Mifflin, 2001, pg. 240.

mind-boggling number of books promise that they "hold the key" and "work," and there are a myriad of pills that "melt the fat away with no exercise or diet." With all these choices, people still waste their money on diet aids. There is now a $32 billion diet and weight loss industry to help people take off the pounds that inevitably result from overindulgence.[6] I ask you, do you really believe these pills or diet books work for the long haul? I am guilty of purchasing ephedra-based products (diet pills containing the Chinese plant ma huang, believed to have a thermogenic, fat burning effect) until I decided to rid myself of my monkey instead. Where has your money gone? (Read, "Are diet pills effective? Fat Chance," *Consumer Reports on Health*, March 2007, www.ConsumerReportsonHealth.org.)

Each year millions of Americans go on diets to lose weight. Most of those millions will experience some degree of weight loss, but only 5 percent or less will keep the fat off permanently. Why? Because, most people view the diet as a temporary change to meet their usually unrealistic goals. Success can only come if you make permanent lifestyle changes. People mindlessly wander down the bookstore aisles in search of the "perfect" weight loss book or meander in the diet store looking for the "magic" pill. I have seen a decade of fad diets and pills cycle through the media with all the hype and marketing available, yet the obesity rate keeps going up. Subsequently, the inevitable happens; the diet comes and goes because of its impracticalities, and everyone waits for the next new "miracle." When is enough, enough? When do you want to gain control of your life? You are the one that decides if you are going to lead a life of overindulgence and poor health or not. I beg you to be in command of your life. Address your monkey and work toward a healthier you. You have the control in your life; even the circumstances that seem beyond your control are still yours to control. We have the power to decide how we are going to react to each moment in our lives. Most people allow the outside influences to control them instead of them being in control. How you personally react to every situation, day in and day

---

6.   Jonathan Rowe, "The Growth Consensus Unravels," *Dollars & Sense The Magazine of Economic Justice*," www.dollarsandsense.org/archives/0799rowe.html, paragraph 18, October 16, 2006.

out, is under your control. Now, take the reins of your life and steer it in the direction *you* choose.

Speaking of choices, we as Americans have chosen to allow our diets to decline, as well as our level of activity. Our society has become sedentary and greatly addicted to the modern conveniences that have dramatically reduced the need for movement. Yet we have not changed our diets to eliminate the calories we once needed to perform simple tasks. I am talking about everything from car washes and remote controls to online shopping. There is little need to exert energy throughout the day because we take the elevator or escalator instead of climbing the stairs. We have power-everything in our cars and moving walkways in our airports. In combination with our desk jobs, these small differences have led to weight gain throughout the years. Don't get me wrong, they are all great conveniences, which I use myself; however, I exercise to ensure I burn extra calories to avoid weight gain. Are you guilty of spending an extra twenty minutes looking for a parking space next to the entrance of a store? Have you ever thought about parking a little further away and walking? Walking—imagine that! Amazingly, so many people do not realize they should be moving more. My intention is not to be mean; I simply want you to start thinking about how your choices affect what you actually want.

Another major element contributing to an overweight America is the size of food portions. In order to attain the goal of well-being, you must be aware of your portion sizes, especially when dining out, and make adjustments. Many people have no concept of a "standard" serving size as defined by the U.S. Department of Agriculture (USDA). From my experience, most restaurants are not either. For example, in the 1950s, a single serving of Coca-Cola was 6.5 ounces; in the 1970s, it was 12 ounces, and by 2000, it had become the 20-ounce bottle.[7] Coca-Cola has increased its single serving size by more than *200 percent* since the 1950s. Fast food restaurants continue to create new supersized items to outdo their competitors. Burger King's *BK Stacker—double, triple or*

---

7.   Gary Gardner and Brian Halweil, "*Overfed and Underfed: The Global Epidemic of Malnutrition,*" Worldwatch Institute, pg. 32.

quad, consist of two, three, or four beef patties and two, three, or four slices of cheese. The *double* weighs in at 610 calories and 39 grams of fat, the *triple* weighs in at 800 calories and 54 grams of fat, and the *quad* weighs in at 1,000 calories and 68 grams of fat.[8] The McDonald's Chicken Selects Premium Breast Strips (10 pc) contains 1,270 calories and 66 grams of fat.[9] Did you know Ruby Tuesday's Colossal Burger weighs in at 1,940 calories and 141 grams of fat? Better yet, you can order one of Uno Chicago Grill's Pizza Skins appetizers that provide approximately 2,050 calories and 48 grams of *saturated* fat.[10] As if we needed more calories! People now consume 42-ounce soft drinks along with their calorie-laden meals. Who on earth needs to be drinking 42 ounces of soda? That is the equivalent of three-and-a-half cans of soda and nearly 600 calories. Even packaged foods have jumped on the super-size bandwagon. Candy bars and potato chips that used to come in 1-ounce servings now come in 2–3 ounce servings. Bagels and muffins that used to be 2–3 ounces are now typically 4–7 ounces. Everything has been "supersized" and is out of control. Are you eating any of these foods?

There is a serious problem when people order a McDonald's Double Quarter Pounder with Cheese, which weighs in at 740 calories and 42 grams of fat, and then they supersize it with an extra-large fries (570 calories and 30 grams of fat) and a 32 ounce Coke (310 calories)—totaling 1,620 calories and 72 grams of fat. This is insanity! What about those of you who order a meal with enough calories for three days, and then ask for a Diet Coke—you are watching your figure, right? Do you find this as upsetting as I do? Unless you are starting to make one small change in your eating habits by switching from regular soda to diet, you have to start taking some responsibility and ask yourself if this is good for you. Take a good look in the mirror, and then try to blame McDonald's or some other fast food restaurant for being overweight or

---

8.   http://www.bk.com/#menu=3,-1,-1, February 26, 2007.

9.   http://www.mcdonalds.com/app_controller.nutrition.index1.html, February 26, 2007.

10.   Jane Hurley and Bonnie Liebman, "X-Treme Eating, increasingly indulgent menus entice diners to pig out," Nutrition Action Healthletter, March 2007, pg. 13.

unhealthy. In the United States, consumers spent about $115 billion on fast food in 2002, more than on higher education or personal computers or new cars.[11] Did you ever think that you are to blame, and that you need to be accountable for your own actions? Wake up! If it is too difficult to enter these places and eat in a healthful way, perhaps you should reconsider going into them. Again, my intention is not to be mean, but rather to have you question yourselves and address what you are doing to yourself.

Need I mention places like The Cheesecake Factory that could feed a family of three with one dinner? While the food may be tasty, the portions are outrageous, and people tend to consume every morsel on their plate—by themselves. The Cheesecake Factory sees value in their portions, which they believe encourages customers to make a second meal of leftovers—really? Howard Gordon, a spokesman for The Cheesecake Factory, said his diners already know how to handle the chain's ample portions.[12]

Food choices and food preparation affect the amount of calories we consume; therefore, be attentive to what and how much you are eating. Numerous studies have found when served more you would eat more. Supersized portions will create supersized people. *Hello*—are you paying attention! Wake up! Please—for the sake of your health.

When you dine out, you do not have as much control of how the dish is prepared. Restaurant food is typically less healthy than home-cooked versions because the meals are usually higher in fat, sodium, and calories. People who eat out more tend to weigh more. Because restaurant food is high in fat and tastes so good, we eat more of it. In addition to the meal itself, most restaurants serve free appetizers such as bread or chips and salsa. Be honest—do you get the breadbasket or chips basket filled up more than once? These calories add up. By consuming the little "extras" before dinner, you could be more than doubling your caloric

---

11.   Diane Martindale, Burgers on the brain, Article from New Scientist vol 177 issue 2380. Date: 1 February 2003.

12.   Daily News Central, "*FDA's Call for Smaller Restaurant Portions Draws Criticism*," June 3, 2006, http://health.dailynewscentral.com/content/view/2279/63, February 20, 2007.

intake. You can simply ask your server not to bring you extras or to remove them—you cannot eat what is not there, right? Perhaps restaurants should offer cheaper half portions, and menus should list the calories for standard meals on the menu.

To make matters worse, food marketing and advertising have increased significantly over the past decade, bombarding the public with messages to convince them to buy and eat more. Food is the most heavily advertised commodity in the United States, and more than half of this advertising is for candy, sweetened breakfast cereals, fast food, and other items of dubious nutritional value.[13] This must be some kind of joke—we are being encouraged to eat more? Do you think we need to be encouraged? We are surrounded by very unhealthy (yes, I know they taste delicious) foods in vending machines, movie theaters, ballparks, restaurants, and convenience stores, all of which exacerbate the problem of reduced movement. We live in a world that promotes unreasonable consumption of high fat, high-calorie foods that are more accessible and cheaper than ever; therefore, we are consuming more calories, moving less, and getting fatter. By surrounding ourselves with higher-calorie foods in oversized portions, we have achieved a predictable result—an oversized society! Maybe our cars have gotten so big because our people have gotten so big.

This availability, affordability, and ease of eating out have contributed greatly to the decline in quality of Americans' diets and the increase in our waistlines. Why order take-out and wait from thirty to forty-five minutes to get the order, when you could spend an equal or lesser amount of time cooking yourself a healthful meal—a meal in which you control the ingredients and therefore its fat, sodium, and overall calories. Homemade food, when prepared with knowledge, can be more nutrient dense and lighter than take-out, and by light, I mean fewer calories. Learn to cook; it can be very simple, especially with the many books and tools available. I usually make meals in less than thirty min-

---

13.   Anthony E. Gallo, "Food Advertising in the United States," in Elizabeth Frazao, ed., *America's Eating habits: Changes and Consequences* (Washington, DC: United States Department of Agriculture (USDA), Economic Research Service (ERS), April 1999.

utes that are healthy and taste great. A home-cooked meal does not mean heating up a pre-packaged meal, eating snack foods, or fast foods. Prepackaged meals are loaded with additives that we should avoid; even many of the healthier premade meals are loaded with sodium—reading the ingredients on some of the pre-packaged meals can get tiring after a while.

Are you healthy from eating this way? Do you feel good? Maybe this has been your lifestyle, so you do not really know what *great* feels like. Has your monkey completely taken over? Take the necessary steps to rid yourself of your monkey, and you will find out how great you can feel when you decide to make choices that support a healthy you, a healthy life. This will not require a complete overhaul. You will simply need to become educated, exercise self-control, and implement healthy alternatives. Most importantly, you must have the real desire to make changes!

True signs that our weight is increasing:

- Because of safety concerns, the Federal Aviation Administration has instructed airlines to add 10 pounds to approved passenger weights.[14]

- Over the last decade, diabetes rates rose 60 percent in the United States.[15]

- Over half of diabetes cases are due to overweight, poor diet and physical inactivity.[16]

- The Gap, Limited Too, and Target are selling plus-sized clothes for youths.[17]

---

14. Phillips D. "Airlines Told to Adjust for Heavier Passengers: FAA Raises Weight Estimates for Safety." *Washington Post*, May 13, 2003, p. A4.

15. Mokdad AH, et al. "Prevalence of Obesity, Diabetes, and Obesity-Related Health Risk Factors, 2001." *Journal of the American Medical Association,* 2003, vol. 289, pp. 76-79.

16. McGinnis JM, Foege WH. "Actual Causes of Death in the United States." *Journal of the American Medical Association,* 1993, vol. 270, pp. 2207-2212. Hu F, et al. "Diet, Lifestyle, and the Risk of Type 2 Diabetes Mellitus in Women." *The New England Journal of Medicine*, 2001, vol. 345, pp. 790-797.

17. Boccella K. "Plus Sizes for Kids Make Way into Stores." *Providence Journal,* March 24, 2002.

- The plus-size clothing market generates $23 billion in sales a year; accounting for a quarter of women's clothing sales.[18]

- One of the reasons that the Boston Red Sox decided to rebuild Fenway Park was that the seats were too narrow for today's baseball fans. The seats in the new ballpark are four inches wider.[19]

Another byproduct of The Land of The Plenty are weight loss surgeries. The number of people undergoing medical procedures such as gastric bypass to help them lose weight greatly concerns me. The procedure is only getting more popular with the assistance of endorsement from celebrities that include Carnie Wilson, Randy Jackson, Al Roker, Rosanne Barr, and Etta James. From 1998 to 2004, the total number of bariatric surgeries increased nine times, from 13,386 to 121,055. National inpatient hospital costs for bariatric surgeries (excluding physician costs) increased by more than eight times from $147 million in 1998 to $1.26 billion in 2004. Nationally, the average cost for a hospital stay for bariatric surgery in 2004 was $10,395. All Americans who pay for health care services share the cost of these surgeries.[20] Increased health premiums affect everyone. For what? Why should people who take responsibility for their health pay for those who do not?

In order to be considered a candidate for weight loss surgery, one must have tried and failed to lose weight through traditional forms of treatment. Individuals hoping to have this surgery go in knowing exactly what to say. I have interviewed six people who have had the surgery and each one of them expressed knowing precisely what to say in order to qualify. Five of the six had to gain additional weight prior to being accepted. In my opinion, many of the people who undergo this type of surgery use it as a last resort because they have never been able to

18. Van Allen P. "Chains to Grow with Plus-Sizes." Philadelphia Business Journal, September 27, 2002.
19. Patton P. "America's Ever-Bigger Bottoms Bedeviling Seating Planners." *Miami Herald*, September 23, 1999.
20. Yafu Zhao, M.S. and William Encinosa, PhD, Bariatric Surgery Utilization and Outcomes in 1998 and 2004, Healthcare cost and utilization project, January 2007, pg.1.

stick to a lifestyle plan. Many of these patients tire of "trying and fail-ing," but neither the patient nor the physician truly addressed their lifestyle issues (bad eating and lack of movement) prior to surgery. Most institutions performing these surgeries do not mandate that the patients undergo nutritional or lifestyle classes pre- or post-surgery. Some classes exist that a patient can *elect* to attend. This is not supportive to those individuals that need this help. Unfortunately, it takes a major medical procedure that *forces* lower calorie consumption for weight reduction to reveal the obvious—fewer calories equals less weight! Most of these people have put the weight on themselves; I believe most of them can take the weight off themselves as well. For the majority of peo-ple who are overweight or obese, I recommend the obvious, decreased caloric intake, increased physical activity, and permanent, healthy lifestyle changes—by prioritizing and making changes one at a time. If you usually sit in front of the TV and eat, start sitting down at the din-ner table and eat—nothing else, just change the environment. Then when eating at the dinner table has become second nature, and you no longer eat while watching TV, and then make another change such as switching your regular coke to diet coke or a flavored low-calorie seltzer. Continue until you have addressed all your unhealthy habits. People have to make the choice and truly *want* to change their behaviors. We are what we repeatedly do.

Surgery for weight reduction is not a miracle procedure. It does not guarantee that you will lose all of your excess weight or that you will keep it off long-term. Weight loss success after gastric bypass surgery depends on your commitment to making lifelong changes in your eat-ing and exercise habits. The reason most people undergo one of these surgeries is because they could not control their eating or they were not exercising, so where is the logic in that? The stomach is a muscular bag that expands and contracts, and as you start to feed it more, little by lit-tle, it has no choice but to expand. The expansion allows for more con-sumption of food, and hence extra calories that lead to weight gain. Would it not be easier and safer to take control of your eating and exer-cise without going under the knife and incurring the associated risks? It is a vicious cycle, but *you* can *gain control of your life and eat properly.* Again, you must truly want to make the necessary changes.

Here is a list of the most common risks specific to weight loss surgeries:

- Depression
- Loss of muscle mass
- Pneumonia
- Protein deficiency
- Transient hair loss
- Vitamin and mineral deficiency

These risks are not as common after weight loss surgeries but are still potential complications:

- Abscess
- Bowel obstruction
- Hemorrhages
- Leakage of bowel connections
- Urinary tract infection
- Wound infection
- One in every two hundred patients die—could you be that one?

A close family friend was on the verge of going under the knife, but instead resolved to make one last attempt at controlling herself and her life by managing her diet and losing the weight. She was able to pinpoint her monkey and make the necessary changes that allowed her to lose over 150 pounds. She continues to work every day to keep her monkey off her back. She has to be very careful and aware of what she eats. Believe me when I tell you that she had tried every diet and pill on the market and had blamed everyone but herself. She finally took a long, hard look at herself and realized that she was the problem and that she needed to manage certain issues. Her monkey was poor self-esteem, which manifested itself through a lack of personal accountability. She was overeating and making poor nutritional choices. She told me that she was consuming nearly *10,000* calories a day. Now she eats between 1,500 and 1,700 calories a day. She also lacked movement in her life. Now her good eating habits have become second nature, and she has changed her life for the better—without surgery—since 2000! To think that she once thought surgery was her only option! So can you, like my friend, get that monkey off your back? I believe you can; now you must believe you can!

Most people's weight problems make them increasingly unhappy. Do you resolve to do better in the morning, only to disappoint yourself? Are you going to hide behind fat clothes instead of making changes? There is no reason to live this way. Follow the written exercises to help rid yourself of your monkey so you can achieve your goals and change your life. You can be in control. Make the choice to be in control!

Taking control can be much easier than you think. For example: do not have a second helping, eat baked instead of fried, use natural peanut butter instead of the brands with added sugar and fat, eat egg whites instead of whole eggs, eat fruit instead of drinking fruit juices, and eat low-fat yogurt or ice cream instead of full fat. Add fibrous vegetables or soups to your meals. Small adjustments like these are extremely effective without turning your life upside down. Do not try to change everything at once; that is a recipe for disaster. Eating should be a joyful and natural experience. If you are inhaling your food, you are not enjoying it, so slow down and take the time to eat and savor.

Do you have the no-carb friend, the no-sugar friend, the no-fat friend? Do any of you have the healthy friend who eats only when she is hungry and does not think about how many calories are in something because she understands good nutrition and portion control? I bet that person will even have dessert occasionally and that she enjoys life without worrying she might gain a pound. Seek out people who are healthy and watch how they eat, what they eat, and how much they eat. You will find your peace with food and be amazed at the freedom that comes from not obsessing about calories, carbs, and so forth. You just have to learn to listen to your body and trust its instincts. Eat real food, not fast food or pre-packaged meals, and do not go hungry.

Whether you are 5 or 50 pounds overweight, telling yourself that you are fat and ugly does not help. Remember, life is full of unpredictable occurrences that are beyond our control, but we do have control over our self-talk. Take control of your mind and begin to take charge of yourself. You have 100 percent control, so use it. Guilt, shame, and blame never lead to positive change. You must speak to yourself about your desire to make changes in a positive way and then hold yourself accountable. Telling yourself you have a keg instead of a six-pack, or that you have cottage cheese thighs, is mean and counterproductive. Make the decision to overcome these negative thoughts and habits. Change today, and then tomorrow, until the change becomes an everyday habit that requires little thought. Remember the exercise "I *am*" followed by what you want to be!

Try to make some real life changes instead of risking your life with surgery, pills, or crazy diets. All surgeries have inherent risks, but the health dangers of gastric reduction surgeries are significant, and complications are common. Diet pills and books can have devastating results as well.

Correspondent Susan Spencer, <u>Doing It The Old-Fashioned Way</u>, September 3, 2004, © MMIV, CBS Worldwide Inc.

Since Seinfeld closed the door on Newman (Wayne Knight) for the last time in 1998, Knight has shed nearly 100 pounds, not through gastric bypass, but the old-fashioned way. He decided to exercise more and eat less.

An obsession with food had plagued him since his childhood in Georgia. And even though he'd made a career in these larger-than-life roles, he realized he had a problem. "I used to have a tan from the light in the refrigerator," says Knight. "I would just know there was something in there that will be the answer." That problem, Knight says, really hit home during a taping of Seinfeld: "I was being fired at by a farmer having been with the farmer's daughter, running through a cornfield with my pants down, and at some point in the middle of shooting, I can't catch my breath." That led to a visit with cardiologist Daniel Eisenberg, who confirmed Knight's worst fears. "I said, 'All the fame in the world isn't going to help you to prevent what most people get, and that's diabetes, heart disease, or strokes.'" "You're heading toward death," says Knight. "And it scared me, literally to life."

Then came the diets. Knight said he went to a bookstore to check out all of the books. But he said he had no interest at all in surgery. It was too scary, and too risky. "I believe that you can eat through a gastric bypass. I believe that, in my previous self, I might have tried," says Knight.

Now, Knight thinks the biggest difference is not being thinner, but being healthier. "I was eating for reasons that have nothing to do with hunger. I was eating to numb myself, and when I began to have to look at the fact that I was eating as an addiction and treat it as such, that's when I turned a corner," says Knight.

Obesity does not affect only adults. Habits start from a young age, and we have adopted most of our habits from the influential people in our lives. Lifestyle habits learned during childhood set the stage for good or poor health in adult life. What you feed your children, and what you yourself eat, will affect your kids for the rest of their lives. Is your child going to be one of the many obese children with countless numbers of medical problems? Doctors are reporting an increase in the number of overweight kids with diabetes, hypertension, and high cholesterol, conditions that used to be largely the province of those middle-aged or older.[21]

Aside from the health risks, the most devastating effects of childhood obesity are the comments, the staring, and the emotional abuse from peers—we have all been kids and we all know how cruel kids can be. It is not a question of *if* someone will tease your child. It is a question of

---

21.   Sandra G. Boodman, "Who are you calling fat?" The Washington Post, July 18, 2006, F1 and F4.

when someone will tease your child. Do you want that for your child? Kids should not be fat, but whose fault is that? Obese children face a poor quality of life. Can you live with that? If not dealt with, this can be scary. Help your child, and do not allow him to develop a monkey. Keep that monkey off his back!

A third of U.S. children and teens—about 25 million kids—are either overweight or on the brink of becoming so.[22] In an article dated July 18, 2006, the *Washington Post* reported that doctors at the Children's National Medical Center in Washington, D.C. treated a nine-year-old who had suffered a heart attack. The child had a Body Mass Index (BMI) of 52. To put that in perspective—an adult standing five foot six inches with a BMI of 52 would weigh 322 pounds. Are you horrified yet? These children are ridiculed and outcast. Do you think these children are the ones chosen for a game of dodge ball or flag football? Even if sports are not your child's thing, you have to realize the harsh emotional and psychological consequences that an overweight child or adolescent will experience when excluded. Please, allow your children a normal, healthy life.

A child's weight is a touchy subject even for most doctors. Many doctors are hesitant to mention a child's weight issues out of fear of alienating the family and hurting the child's feelings. Childhood obesity is out of control. Many overweight children have overweight parents who are reluctant to make changes themselves, and as a result, their child suffers. These children are at a risk of developing life-threatening illnesses before the age of twenty. Playing the "mean" parent and saying no to candy and fast food will not seem so bad when your child is battling heart disease. It gets more difficult to teach healthful habits as a child gets older. Give your child the opportunity to lead a healthy life. Additionally, parents that keep snacks and junk foods usually consume them as well; therefore, you would be doing yourself a favor by eliminating these types of foods and replacing them with healthier alternatives.

---

22.   Nanci Hellmich, "Third of kids tip the scales the wrong way," USA Today, April 15, 2006.

According to a recent national study by Harvard Medical School, ten-to fifteen-year-old boys spend, on average, three-and-a-half hours a day watching television or playing video games, and girls the same age spend two-and-a-half hours on average doing the same thing. Children are typically in school for eight hours and sleep for eight hours, so when are your children moving?

If you are overweight, the probability is good that your child will be overweight. Children pick up the habits demonstrated to them. This is usually not an issue of genetics, but instead, their environment. If you feel your child's weight problem is the result of a medical condition, please visit your child's pediatrician. However, chances are good that the issue has more to do with lifestyle, poor nutrition, and inactivity.[23] The incidence of childhood obesity has approximately doubled over the last two decades; however, genetic characteristics have not changed during that time. When was the last time you went for a walk, let alone participated in a full-fledged workout? Your children mimic you, so blame yourself. *Do not* blame the fast food industry, video games, television, computers, or the lack of physical education in schools! Of course, all these things have exacerbated the situation, but you must take responsibility for yourself and your children. You must set an example!

23. Sharon Mickle, "Snacks, Sodas—and Calories—Climbing in Kids," Food Surveys Research Group, http://www.ars.usda.gov/is/np/fnrb/fnrb1000.htm, February 21, 2007.

Table 4:

Start making some incremental changes:

- **Assess <u>your</u> own habits and health.** Be honest with yourself first, and then work together as a family for a common goal.

- **Involve your children.** Work together as a family, because the home environment is one of the strongest influences on behavior. If your children see you moving more and eating well, you will set a positive image for them to emulate.

- **At mealtimes, offer children whatever you are eating,** instead of "kid food" (easy-to-prepare child pleasers like pizza, macaroni and cheese, and chicken nuggets). Learn how to make healthier alternatives to their favorite foods. Be creative.

- **Get your children to eat breakfast.** By breakfast, I do not mean a sausage, egg, and cheese biscuit from McDonald's. Breakfast should be a healthful meal such as whole grain toast and milk, high fiber cereals (not Captain Crunch), oatmeal and blueberries (not Pop Tarts). Teach your children the right habits.

- **You do not have to forbid fast food;** just do not make it a big part of your children's lives, and do not reward them with it either. There are far better rewards than food for good grades or behavior. Let them know the benefits of nutritional eating.

- **Keep healthy snacks in the house.** Ditch the soda and candy and opt for healthier choices like fruit, nuts, and air-popped popcorn. If you want to keep juices in the house, make sure they are 100 percent juice without any added sugar or preservatives. Cut up vegetables and have low-fat string cheese. There are so many alternatives to high fat, high sugar, highly processed foods. Give your children healthy options.

- **Encourage your children to help you with food preparation.** I loved watching my parents cook, and now, I love to cook. Since my parents were health conscious, I am as well. Involve your children in the kitchen and allow them to learn.

- **Sit down at the table, not in front of the TV, and eat as a family.** Families that eat together develop better dietary habits. Create a positive environment with regard to food and meals. Your focus should be on your meal and each other. Learn about each other, and enjoy one another's company. Mindless eating has become far too common. TV is a distraction and causes many people to overeat. I also encourage you to serve everyone and then put the food away, because you are less likely to serve yourself or your children seconds if it requires a deliberate effort on your part. Keeping food on the table allows for mindless eating.

- **Get your children involved with cleanup.** They can help clear the table, wash the dishes, and clean the kitchen. Not only are they moving a little, they are also learning responsibility.

- **Control your child's school lunches.** The nutritional quality of most school lunches is below average and poor. There are many organizations devoted to adding healthier alternatives including vegetarian fare. Become involved and recommend alternatives. You can lobby to change the items in the vending machines or even the hot lunches, but do something. You can influence this situation. Send your child with a lunch that you have prepared with nutritional knowledge and love. Visit http://www. knowledgenetwork.ca/makingithappen/.

- **For the health and well-being of your children, turn off the TV, games, and computers, and get your child moving.** Do not allow your children to have a television in their bedroom. If they already have one, remove it immediately.

- **If you are not moving, your children probably are not either.** If you move, they will move. Play catch with your children, teach them to ice skate, roller skate, or ride a bike, and get them involved in athletics. Do not let your children sit at school all day, then come home and sit in front of the TV eating chips. Use your common sense, and do what is right for your children!

Being knowledgeable on nutrition and moving more are two of the most important things you can do for yourself and your family. Healthy eating cannot be a part-time or temporary thing. As a society, we must recognize that what we have been doing is not working. We are making people rich by buying into their diet frauds and "magic" BS pills. Do not throw your money away—invest in your health instead by educating yourself and your family. Stop making people rich who are selling products that compromise your health and quality of life. Please, save your money and *eat that monkey instead*!

We, as a society have developed a bad habit of misplacing blame. We hold the fast food companies responsible for making us fat even though they do not make you go in, buy their food, and eat it. As I stated before, the food industry is second only to the automobile industry in advertising, and they have spent their money well because they have the consumer hook, line, and sinker. However, instead of taking responsibility for our actions and ourselves, we blame "others" for our obesity while continuing to give them our business. Do we not care about our health and well-being, or are we weak-minded and allow ourselves to fall prey to their marketing efforts and stay unhealthy? Things that make you go *hmmmmmmmm*.

I am giving you the guidelines that you need to overcome this *reversible* problem. It will take your commitment and dedication. Take an extensive look at yourself and allow the time to make the necessary changes in a manner that is healthy and controllable. You have to give yourself the freedom to live life to its fullest. However, you have to *want* to make a change. *Only you can do it!*

Become part of a healthy America by eating your monkey!

Chapter Five

Do You Really Need to Lose Weight?

"There's only one corner of the universe you can be certain of improving, and that's your own self."
~Aldous Huxley

"Our greatest glory is not in never failing, but in rising up every time we fail."
~Ralph Waldo Emerson

"You hold the greatest power of all: the ability to design your own life. It's what you decide to do each morning and how you feel at the end of the day. It's choosing to ignore limitations and being open to life's possibilities. All of them. It's your mind, body and spirit—your journey."
Ready to Exercise your Options?
~February 2001 Fitness Magazine (Anonymous)

Extra pounds weigh you down, put added stress on the body and organs, can throw off your hormones, and put you at a higher risk for diabetes, hypertension, sleep apnea, depression (and other emotional issues), heart disease, fertility problems, and countless other obesity-related illnesses and conditions. Do you suffer from any of these health problems? How is your energy level? Are you able to climb a flight of stairs without a problem? Do your joints ache due to extra weight? If you answered *yes* to any of these questions, now is the time to change your life!

Do you love yourself for who you are? Do you treat yourself in a respectful manner? Do you agree that making your health a priority is loving and respectful of yourself? The first requirement for a happy existence on this planet is to love the person you are morally and ethically; however, I believe that if you truly love yourself, you would not jeopardize your health. If you are putting your health at risk, you had better open your eyes and do something about it. It is your body and your responsibility. Do you want to live a life of aches, pains, and health problems? Are you truly happy with yourself? You have the choice to live a remarkable life in good health. Do not deny yourself optimal health.

Not being at your healthy weight can adversely affect your life. You will not be physically capable of participating in activities that you want or need to do, and you may become so preoccupied with your weight that you shy away from things that you really would like to do. Are you willing to accept less from the only life you get? Working toward your healthy weight will allow you to work toward happiness and a better quality of life.

Do not obsess over the "perfect number" on the scale; shooting for some fantasy number is counterproductive. Consult with a preventative medicine doctor, dietician, internist, or nutritionist to find out what your healthy weight range should be. Everyone is a different size and shape, so find out what *your* true size and shape are. You cannot change your short torso, long legs, short legs, big feet, or whatever else you might dwell on. *Accept the things that are uniquely yours and work from there.* Focus on being a healthier you, as opposed to what size clothes you can wear.

Fat is not you—you can get rid of it. Just because you have yet to be successful does not mean the weight is yours to keep. You must analyze yourself and figure out what your monkey is and take the time to make the healthful changes necessary to improve your life. There are no "miracles" or "quick fixes."

You will be amazed at the number of positive changes that will occur when you start to eat and exercise for a healthier you. For example, The Diabetes Prevention Program found that a mere 7 percent drop in weight—*7 percent!*—along with increased physical activity could delay or even prevent Type II diabetes in high-risk patients. You will also be surprised at how much better you will feel after dropping 7 percent of your weight. Let me put that into perspective: if you weigh 200 pounds, you would only need to lose 14 pounds to start benefiting.

Do not be discouraged, because you truly have more control than you think. Your genes are roughly 33 percent responsible for your shape and size, which means that the environment serves as the principal influence over your weight. This is obvious when you consider the dramatic increase in body weight and obesity in the last decade. Therefore, while genes do have an impact on the body, especially for people with such conditions as Prader-Willi syndrome[1] and hypothyroidism[2], your environment ultimately determines how fat you become. The food and lifestyle choices you make truly are what shape your life. While the women in your family may have a larger hip-to-waist ratio, or the men in your family have spare tires, this is not your destiny. Fat is not you. *Unhealthy* is a choice—a choice that is usually learned—but one that can certainly be changed. Now you must alter these bad habits and implement healthy ones. You can reshape and mold your body into a healthy, strong one through exercise and mindful eating.

---

1. Medline Plus Medical Encyclopedia, http://www.nlm.nih.gov/medlineplus/ency/article/001605.htm, February 21, 2007.
2. Medline Plus Medical Encyclopedia, http://www.nlm.nih.gov/medlineplus/ency/article/000353.htm, February 21, 2007.

There are incentives out there for you to take control of your life—use them! Check with your insurance provider or speak to your primary care physician to find out whether medical nutritional therapy (visits with a dietician or nutritionist) is covered. *Get that monkey off your back and begin your new and improved life!*

Correspondent Richard Schlesinger, "The Subway Diet" September 3, 2004, © MMIV, CBS Worldwide Inc.

(CBS) Jared Fogle, 26, is best known as "The Subway Guy," after the brand of sandwiches that he says helped him lose 245 pounds in a year …

… Six years ago, as a junior at Indiana University, Jared weighed a staggering 425 pounds …

… Growing up in Indianapolis, Jared was the only one in his family with a weight problem. "Food was a comfort to me. It replaced personal relationships. It replaced extracurricular activities. It replaced everything in my life," says Jared.

How was he able to carry that weight around? "It's very difficult. It hurts. My shoulders would hurt. My knees would hurt. My wrists would hurt," says Jared. "And that was not even when I was in motion."

For years, his parents tried to get him to eat right. His father, who was also his doctor, knew that Jared would experience severe health problems if he didn't change. But by the time he was 20, Jared was eating enough for five people—sometimes, 10,000 calories a day.

Consider what Jared was consuming…. Every day for breakfast, he'd have two bacon, egg and cheese sandwiches, with a large order of hash browns, a large coffee with cream and 10 packets of sugar.

Lunch was an entire pizza—extra meat, extra cheese, and of course dessert. Believe it or not, he would need a mid-afternoon snack—usually two large bean burritos with extra cheese.

And dinner? That usually consisted of not one or two, but three trips to the Chinese buffet, and ice cream for dessert.

Then, he topped off each day with a late-night snack—not a warm glass of milk, but usually a hamburger, French fries and some kind of dessert. It's not easy consuming 10,000 calories every single day.

Before he started controlling his weight, he says his weight was controlling him: "Whereas most college students pick their classes on the teacher, or the class itself, or the time of day, for me it was, did they have adequate seating that could fit me in that particular classroom?"

It got so bad that just walking across campus became a daily struggle for Jared. "I would take steps, but then I'd have to, maybe every 20 steps or so, I'd have to catch my breath."

Jared knew the time had come to lose weight, but the first several attempts failed …

… Soon, he cut his daily consumption from 10,000 calories a day to just 2,000.

"This was a major change. I mean, not to make a pun, but I dieted cold turkey," says Jared.

Most people don't even weigh 245 pounds, much less lose that much. But in just one year, Jared dropped from 425 pounds to a relatively svelte 190 pounds—a weight he has now maintained for five years.

Chapter Six

Pardon Me While I Laugh

"Anything worth having is not easy.... If it were easy, everyone would do it."
~Anonymous

Ready to Exercise Your Options?
~Fitness Magazine, February 2001

"Never, never, never give up."
~Winston Churchill

Where does one start with the inestimable number of "diets" that are *guaranteed* to work. Who guarantees them? Did you ever think that if there are so many diet books, that maybe they do not work? Some of you may have lost some weight, but the real question is, have you managed to keep it off? You haven't? I'm sure you must have done something wrong (I happen to be a very sarcastic individual)! Did you adhere to all the "rules"? It's not you. These diets set you up for success only to push you back down and create feelings of despair and failure.

Nearly all diets fail because people resume their previous eating habits. People repeat and abandon the diet many times, and most see an overall increase in their weight. Yo-yo dieting is just that: your weight and self-esteem go up and down. Fad diets and pills come and go, but the basic concepts behind reaching and keeping a healthy weight are realistic and unchanging. The "weight loss" industry relies on the ignorance of the public and so far, they have played us for fools. The diet industry continues to expand, as do our waistlines. Another day, another diet. Sound familiar? Desperate? These books are not addressing the real issue—your monkey. They fail to encourage permanent and realistic changes. The list is endless, and I would have to have a separate book to name all of the ridiculous diet plans that have come and gone.

Here are just a few of the diets that have been, or are currently, on the market:

- *Atkins, New Diet Revolution*
- *Dr. Phil's Diet Plan*
- *Mayo Clinic Diet*
- *Optifast Diet*
- *Ornish*
- *Pritikin*
- *Sugar Busters*
- *Suzanne Somers' "Somersizing" Plan*
- *The Abs Diet*
- *The All-You-Can-Eat Soup Diet*

- *The Blood Type Diet*
- *The Cabbage Soup Diet*
- *The Chili Pepper Diet*
- *The Fast Food Diet*
- *The Fat Flush Plan*
- *The Grapefruit Diet, Liquid Diets, Greenwich Diet*
- *The Hormone Revolution Weight-Loss Plan*
- *The Rice Diet*
- *The Scarsdale Diet*
- *The Shangri-La Diet*
- *The Sonoma Diet*
- *The South Beach Diet*
- *The T-Factor Diet*
- *The Zone*
- *The 3-Hour Diet*
- *The 5-Day Miracle Diet*

Any crash diet deprives your body of the essential nutrients it needs to function properly. Restricting calories causes the loss of not only fat, but also your precious muscle. Muscle is active tissue that requires calories just to exist. Since muscle is tight and compact, and fat is the opposite, muscle looks much better—so why would you want to jeopardize muscle? A nutritionally sound diet along with exercise is the key to maintaining appropriate bodyweight and health.

The USDA and its Human Nutrition Research Centers have launched a new initiative to address what the USDA calls the "long-neglected need for rigorous research on popular diets." There are no efficacy or safety tests for many of these diets. Therefore, I think it is important for you to know a few things about these diet plans.

The Chili Pepper Diet claims that the chili is the missing link in low-fat diets. Some people believe that Capsaicin, the substance that makes a chili *hot*, can improve one's health by increasing blood circulation and metabolism. The author states she did not feel hungry or deprived on her diet, and neither did she feel the need to cheat. The diet does not allow much in the way of food variety, and science certainly has not been able to conclude that capsaicin has any relevance on aiding weight loss. One thing is sure: you would have to consume boatloads of this spice for any metabolic enhancement power. Again, this diet is not practical or sustainable. No single food exists that aids in weight loss. If this were the case, everybody would be devouring chili peppers all day long. Add chili peppers to a well-balanced diet because of their health benefits, not their speculated weight-loss ability.

Detox diets are supposed to rid the body of toxins to help you lose weight. Most detox diets are nutritionally unsound and do not provide sufficient calories. They are essentially fasts. The body has its own detoxification system already. Your liver, kidneys, respiratory and gastrointestinal systems work together to detoxify the body every day. If there really is a problem with your body detoxifying itself, you do not need one of these diets, you need a doctor, because you could have a serious medical condition. Avoid diets that promise to cleanse, purify, or detoxify the body. You can eliminate most problems within the body by consuming whole foods and removing processed foods from your diet. What difference would a cleanse make if you immediately return to your prior unhealthy ways? The intentions of these diets are good, as long as they are a way of life, consuming sufficient calories on a daily basis.

The Grapefruit Diet was first introduced in the 1920s. It promised dieters that they would slim down in approximately three weeks. The catch—you would only eat the "fat burning fruit." People lost weight because they ate about 800 calories a day. To this day, there is no scientific evidence that grapefruit has any fat burning qualities. Do you think this is a diet for you? Excuse me while I laugh!

Where do I start with *The Fat Flush Plan*? It states that you can actually flush out fat by forgoing some foods and eating others. Wow—I did not know it was that simple. In the preface, it reads, "There are no quick fixes—but *The Fat Flush Plan* comes close." It is "a quick and easy way to erase those pockets of fat." She even states that she will be there to help you. I bought the book, and she still has not shown up or called me. On this diet, you eliminate the "evil whites": white sugar, white rice, white bread, and pasta. I was not aware that a low-fat food like rice caused people to get fat. Somebody should tell the Asians. The World Health Organization reports that in Japan, just 1.8 percent of men and 2.6 percent of women have a body mass index above 30. A score of 30 on the BMI is the cutoff for obesity. However, more than 20 percent of men and nearly 25 percent of women in the United States are obese. The Japanese eat rice and vegetables. The difference is that they are not eating every meal as if it is their last supper. The bottom line is that you have to consume fewer calories than the body uses to cause a caloric deficit, and then you will see the fat come off. Quite simply—it is a myth to think that certain foods will flush out fat.

On to Atkins. The release of *Dr. Atkins' Diet Revolution* was in 1972, and Dr. Atkins' New Diet Revolution in 1992 and 1999 followed it. Dr. Atkins published a final addition in 2002. It had few changes, except he did not miss the opportunity to expand his empire by including another moneymaking scheme: by eating this way, you must use vitamin supplements, and since he created the diet, you should buy your supplements from him. Genius! He was a master marketeer! In my opinion, and in the opinion of many scientists and doctors around the world, the Atkins Diet is anything but health promoting. More than 10 million people have followed the Atkins diet (there were more than 10 million copies sold and I'm sure, as I do with most of my books, people shared), and still obesity rates are climbing.

The first two weeks on Atkins are the "induction" period; during this time, dieters eat no more than 20 grams of carbohydrates a day (a banana has more carbs). You are restricted to a diet consisting of nearly unlimited meats, poultry, seafood, eggs, cheeses, oils, butter, bacon, and sausages (as long as they are not cured with sugar). After the first two weeks, dieters begin adding more carbs: five more grams of carbohydrates weekly. When dieters reach the maintenance phase, their diet will generally consist of no more than 40–90 grams of carbohydrates (roughly a bowl of oatmeal and a banana). Sound like a diet you would enjoy for the long haul? Since when did eating fruits like apples, bananas, oranges, grapes, or mangos make people fat? There is *no* scientific data in medical literature supporting that a well-balanced diet that includes a moderate amount of carbohydrates will make you fat.

Last time I checked the foods that are helping ward off cancers and various other illnesses are not steak and butter. On the contrary—they are fruits such as blueberries, oranges, and grapes, and vegetables such as broccoli, asparagus, and onions, along with whole grains and oats— most of the foods that Atkins has you completely avoid because he says they make you fat. Could it be that you are simply eating too many calories? Please, take a moment right now and consider the true absurdity of the Atkins proposition. Great. Now think about it for another moment. Keep thinking about it until you want to yell at someone for actually printing it.

The Physicians Committee for Responsible Medicine (http://www. pcrm.org), a leading advocate for preventive medicine—especially good nutrition—brings you AtkinsDietAlert.org. PCRM has been speaking out about the dangers of high-protein, low-carbohydrate diets since its founding in 1972. "Scientific studies show that low-carbohydrate diets raise cholesterol levels in a considerable number of individuals, sometimes to a dramatic degree. In addition, low-carb diets typically accelerate calcium loss—this has led major health organizations to raise important questions regarding their connection in contributing to heart problems, kidney abnormalities, osteoporosis, and other health problems. Given the seriousness of these health risks, and the strength of the scientific evidence currently available, PCRM hopes it will encourage people to be wary of high-protein diets and to choose healthier options."

The term "low-carb" has no legal definition, and neither do "net-carb" or "effective-carb," despite the free use of these terms on labels and in supermarkets—it is simply great marketing at work. Low-carbohydrate diets typically include quantities of cholesterol, fat, saturated fat, and protein that exceed the recommended safe limits set by the National Academy of Sciences (www.nationalacademies.org) and the USDA (www.usda.gov). They are also lower in fiber and other important dietary components. The Nutrition Committee of the Council on Nutrition, Physical Activity, and Metabolism of the American Heart Association states, "High-protein diets are not recommended because they restrict healthful foods that provide essential nutrients and do not provide the variety of foods needed to adequately meet nutritional needs. Individuals who follow these diets are, therefore, at risk for compromised vitamin and mineral intake, as well as potential cardiac, renal, bone, and liver abnormalities overall."

Let us look at *The South Beach Diet. The South Beach Diet must* be a worthwhile diet; it did after all sell millions of copies and was the number two best seller of 2004 (*The Da Vinci Code* was number one). It just goes to show that the never-ending search for the diet that works is a search by many. Take comfort in the fact that you are not alone. Remember, *The South Beach Diet* came out after Atkins, and Atkins was supposedly the final answer to solving people's weight problems. This diet, along with countless other diet programs, uses phases similar to Atkins. The first fourteen days do not allow bread, rice, potatoes, pasta, baked goods, or even fruit. I cannot take this nonsense any longer, can you? By now, Americans ought to know that just because something sells well, does not mean it is worth buying. Yet the flawed logic prevails.

The major reason *The South Beach Diet* or any other diet book has been so successful is that their publishers have spent millions of dollars to promote these books. A marketing budget equal to theirs could turn a dishwasher repair manual into a major best seller. I suspect that most people who purchase one of these "diet" books care much more about the weight loss aspect than they do about bettering their health. Most diets have very little to do with improving your health and can lead you in the opposite direction. What are you really trying to change or resolve? *Make the choice* to change your life by improving your overall well-being.

Some foods are more nutritionally sound and provide greater health benefits than others, but when you learn *moderation*, you will be able to enjoy *all* the foods you love. For weight loss, these books might work for some in the short-term, but most people will not keep the weight off. In addition to the bad practices and habits these books encourage, there is another reason we fail with these plans: psychology. Undoubtedly, the main reason most people will fail at losing weight permanently on most of these popular diets is that they offer no real solutions for the emotional challenges that come with people's normal eating habits, and much less those associated with dieting. The emotional challenges are usually greater than knowing the rights and wrongs of eating. The written exercises from chapters 1 and 3 are real solutions to the emotional challenges (your monkey) such as cravings, food addictions, self-image issues, and other self-sabotaging behaviors. You must take responsibility for yourself and learn what your monkey is so that you are capable and prepared to handle and resolve the psychological issues perpetuating your weight problem. It is OK, and I encourage you, to seek out the additional help of other people and/or professionals. You must get that monkey off your back, or you will revert to your old habits. Let go of the typical "diet death spiral"!

This dieting roller coaster confuses the body, the metabolism, and the mind. Please be aware that the physical consequences of dieting are just one danger—there is also the psychological aspect of repeated failure. Most diets are one-size-fits-all and "one-size-fits-all" completely ignores the fact that we are *individuals* with different genetic requirements for optimal health—individuals with different tastes, different likes and dislikes, individuals who are vegetarians or vegans, and individuals with different food tolerances. When your diet becomes nutritionally sound, you will understand that these "diets" are nothing more than gimmicks. Please, for the sake of your health, eat fruits, vegetables, and whole grains. Have a sandwich if that is what you would like. You have to become educated on this subject, or you will lose the battle of the bulge. I promise you, more "miraculous" weight loss books and pills will come out, and yes, some will work for a week or two. However, when some people get off the diet, they will be heavier than before. When you veer off one of these one-size-fits all diets, even just a little bit, it's over, and so are your weight loss efforts. I know that I want a body I can be proud of day in and day out for the rest of my life, not for just one event to impress someone. Change your life for good and get off this dangerous roller coaster. Stop the madness and learn to eat for life. *Eat that monkey*!

Our thought process and our unresolved emotions are usually the culprits that cause us to keep those extra pounds. Use the written exercises in the book to help you change harmful habits and resolve to live a healthy life. For example, do you eat even when not physically hungry? This emotional eating will prevent you from losing weight until you face yourself and the real underlying issues—your monkey. When most people begin a weight loss program, they cut out comfort foods, and when drastically reducing or eliminating these foods, your "monkey" emotions have a tendency to surface. If you do not deal with the real issues, no diet will ever work. You have to address *why* you are overeating. You must determine what is eating you! You *can choose* to *change* your life.

Better health is a *choice*, not a two-week gimmick. Permanent weight loss requires either consuming fewer calories through diet alone or through the combination of diet and exercise—not by cutting out whole food groups. Life already has so many rules and regulations—do not complicate it even further. You do not have to entirely eliminate any food, especially if it's something you enjoy. You must learn the fine art of moderation! Most importantly, whatever you do, please, *do not* starve yourself!

Supplements and pills that promise you weight loss are losing you money, not weight. *Nothing can take the place of proper nutrition and exercise.* By incorporating a nutritional philosophy that you can maintain for life—one that focuses on nutrient-dense, unprocessed foods— you can and will change your life. In addition, integrate some form of cardiovascular exercise (movements that get your heart racing, blood pumping, skin sweating, and lungs panting) and weight training (free-weight lifting, weight machines, or anything that safely strains your muscles, ligaments, and bones to grow stronger) into your life, and you will be amazed at your increased vigor and strength. The workouts will assist in burning calories and help you lose or maintain your weight, but most notably, they will improve your overall health and well-being.

We all have our weak moments—a piece of cheesecake here, and a missed workout there—but these are not diet disasters. *It is not the mistake itself that hurts your weight loss efforts, it is how you react to your mistakes.* It's OK; just get back on track. If your energy intake exceeds your energy output, you will gain weight—it's that simple. *Do not cheat yourself! Reward yourself! Get that monkey off your back!*

Chapter Seven

If You Lose, They Lose—
Why Some People Want You Fat

"If we want to change the quality of our lives, we must change what we
habitually ask of ourselves and others."
~Anthony Robbins

"Enjoy the grass on your side of the fence!"
~Author Unknown

"We come to feel as we behave."
~Paul Pearsali

Keeping you fat is economically beneficial. Sales of prescription medicines worldwide are approximately $602 billion, according to IMS health, a pharmaceutical information and consulting company. The United States accounts for the lion's share of this, with $252 billion in annual sales. Most pharmaceutical companies have drugs related to health issues associated with an unhealthy lifestyle and/or increased weight issues. These drugs include, but are not limited to, drugs for cholesterol, blood pressure, hypertension and diabetes, and they are extremely profitable. These drugs are up there with the pain management, sexual enhancement, and depression markets. Pfizer's cholesterol pill Lipitor remains the best-selling drug in the world for the fifth year in a row. Its annual sales in 2006 were $12.9 billion.[1]

Unfortunately, the pharmaceutical companies must do whatever is in their power to keep these profits up, including putting pressure on the Federal Drug Administration (FDA). Let me remind you of drugs such as Vioxx that should never have been put on the market or, at the very least, should have been pulled much sooner. The pharmaceutical companies are always eager to squeeze out more profit, even if patients are having medical complications.[2] The evidence is astounding and the number of articles dedicated to this topic is endless. I invite you to do a search for yourself.

Drug profits are up; are we any healthier because of it? Many people suffer from the toxic side effects of taking just one medication. What about those of you who are taking a combination of several different prescriptions? Statistics show that prescription drugs are killing thousands of Americans each year and causing severe side effects to millions of others. Adverse drug reactions (ADRs) may be the fourth to sixth

1.   Matthew Herper and Peter Kang, "The World's 10 Best Selling Drugs," Forbes.com, March 28, 2006.
2.   Ritt Goldstein, "Drug Industry Scandal a 'Crisis,'" Inter Press Service News Agency, Oct. 4, 2004 and Ashley Pringle (under Supervision from Dr. Chris McDonald, "Pharmaceutical Scandal or not? The Distinction Elaborated," www.pharmacoethics.com/categorization.html, February 21, 2007 and Mike Adams, "Merck now under criminal investigation by the Justice Department for Vioxx scandal," NewsTarget.com, January 1, 2005.

leading cause of death. Serious ADRs occur in 6.7 percent of hospital-ized patients.[3] Your health is far more important than shareholder ben-efits!

Another alarming fact is that since the FDA allowed direct-to-con-sumer advertising in the late 1990s, drug firms have spent billions of dollars in advertising on television and in magazines and newspapers. The advertising has paid off because many consumers enter their doc-tor's offices demanding the medications they see advertised. Many times that is precisely what the doctors prescribe. Additionally, the U.S. press has had mixed feelings when it comes to any negative reporting of drug companies (or their products) because they are benefiting from the drug advertising money. Have you ever heard the phrase, "don't bite the hand that feeds you"? (I highly recommend you read "Death by Medicine," by Gary Null, PhD; Carolyn Dean MD, ND; Martin Feldman, MD; Debora Rasio, MD; and Dorothy Smith, PhD.)

This issue is real. Many of the diseases that plague people have natu-ral remedies. If we remain unhealthy and dependent upon medications such as Lipitor then profits stay high. After all, money is power, and power is money. This is happening at the expense of your health. If you became healthy and lost weight to control issues such as diabetes, cho-lesterol, high blood pressure, or hypertension, sales for these drugs would go down. They would lose the profit and they would lose the power. This can change with you—you can take the power back! You do not have to rely on prescription drugs as a means of well-being. Start asking what alternatives you have. If you are taking medications, consult with your physician and ask if you can make adjustments through lifestyle related changes.

The purpose of this chapter is to inform you so that you can begin to ask questions, the answers to which may have a direct impact on your health. Can lifestyle changes have an impact on your health, thus limit-ing or omitting the use of drugs? Why does your doctor prescribe one

---

3.   American Heart Association, "Statistics you need to know-Statistics on Medication," http://www.americanheart.org/presenter.jhtml?identifier=107, February 21, 2007 (Source for medication statistics: The National Council on Patient Information and Education).

medication over another? Does your doctor talk to you about your lifestyle? Would you take your doctor's advice regarding lifestyle? Are you taking prescription medications? Keep reading and ask yourself these same questions at the end of the chapter.

Do ethics ever get in the way of making a good, healthy profit?[4] Scientists and individuals with direct financial conflicts of interest sit on pharmaceutical advisory committees. The Center for Science in the Public Interest (CSPI) found that of thirty-two experts serving on the FDA's Arthritis Drug and Drug Safety Advisory Committee, ten had received funding from Pfizer, Merck, or Novartis. Pfizer makes Celebrex and Bextra, Merck makes Vioxx, and Novartis is developing a similar drug. At the end of the three-day meeting designed to assess the cardio-vascular risk presented by these drugs, the panel voted to keep these drugs on the market. According to *The New York Times*, the committee would have recommended that Bextra and Vioxx be withdrawn were it not for the votes of scientists with conflicts. (I recommend you read the excerpt from Jonathan Cohn's "Medicare Reform: The Real Winners, TNR: Insurance Companies, Drug Manufacturers Come out Ahead," in the notes section at the end of the book.)

Many sales reps, regardless of profession, have budgets for wining and dining clients—pharmaceutical sales reps are no exception. Can ham on rye influence what a physician prescribes?[5] Regretfully, there is a chance that a pharmaceutical company has compromised your doctors' objectivity. Start to ask questions and do research so that you can have the quality of life that you deserve. What changes can you make that you have control over—prevention through lifestyle?

I have had numerous conversations with people in regards to their doctors prescribing medications without ever asking about the individual's lifestyle habits. There is something very wrong with this! I have a very close friend whose cholesterol diagnosis was high. His doctor pre-

---

4. Jonathan Cohn, "Medicare Reform: The Real Winners, TNR: Insurance Companies, Drug Manufacturers Come Out Ahead," The New Republic Story, Nov. 20, 2003.

5. Stephanie Saul, "Drug makers pay for lunch as they pitch," *The New York Times*, July 28, 2006, C1 and C7.

scribed one of the many statin drugs on the market. Prior to the diagnosis, my friend lived a sedentary life, and his diet was full of saturated fats and nutritionally hollow foods. When he left his doctor's office, he was concerned enough about his situation to do a little research. He had reached the conclusion that he would not take the medication, and instead he opted to exercise to lose weight. His diet remained relatively unchanged, but he was significantly more active than he had been previously. When he returned to the doctor for his follow up, his cholesterol was 100 percent normal—from exercise alone. This motivated him to eat even better and have more respect for his health and life. He wants to be around for his grandchildren and perhaps even his grandchildren's children. My friend still watches his diet and works out regularly. He has maintained a healthy cholesterol level, without drugs. Why did his doctor prescribe a medication and not recommend weight loss and better eating habits to begin with? You have the right to ask these questions. When are we going to become a society focused on prevention? You can correct many underlying imbalances by making changes to your lifestyle, particularly your nutrition and exercise habits.

Prescription drugs used for any illness have many side effects that can include birth defects, neurological disorders, and even death.[6] These are more reasons to try to reduce or eliminate symptoms of obesity through natural and healthful habits. Prescription drugs *are, in many cases,* necessary. They have improved the lives of millions. However, when it comes to the issues you can deal with through lifestyle changes and sometimes weight loss, these drugs are spoiling the quality of life for hundreds of thousands of people, and in extreme cases, causing premature deaths. Not to mention all the costs associated with these prescriptions and medical visits.

I believe that for the most part, many of these drugs are unnecessary and are overprescribed. As a nation, we need to start making changes

---

6.   Maryann Napoli, "Many Prescription Drugs Have Unexpected Harmful Effects," *Center for Medical Consumers, Inc.*, May 2002. Gary Null PhD, Carolyn Dean MD ND, Martin Feldman MD, Debora Rasio MD, Dorothy Smith PhD, "Death by Medicine," 2003, entire document.

through healthful habits, not drugs. Remember, each of us has the power to choose—choose health. You can relieve many of the ailments that stem from extra weight or obesity by making changes in diet and exercise. In many cases, there are no real benefits from these drugs, given that they do not deal with the root of the problem. What exactly are the side effects of diet and exercise? Better health! Now, before you go and get your panties in a bunch—I have not said in *all* cases. I am very aware of the benefits of modern science and medicine, when their needs are true. (Take a look at the Physicians Committee for Responsible Medicine (PCRM) http://www.pcrm.org/ and *The Side Effects Bible: The Dietary Solution to Unwanted Side Effects of Common Medications* by Frederic Vagnini, MD and Barry Fox, PhD).

Are you getting the quality health care you deserve? Regrettably, many patients do not get quality medical care at all. What you do get are drugs. When you visit your doctor, is the waiting room full of people? Do you have to wait beyond your appointment time? Does your doctor really communicate with you? Does he spend enough time with you? My experience has been that many doctors spend *maybe* five minutes with you before making a diagnosis, prescribing pills, and sending you on your way. Does this sound or feel familiar? Has your doctor asked you any questions related to the life you lead outside his office that could have an impact on your well-being? You can change this. Make a list prior to going to the doctor, ask questions, and demand time! Please, be honest with your doctor—tell the truth—if you are a smoker, how much do you smoke? What are you eating? How much exercise are you getting? What prescriptions are you taking? Which vitamins are you taking? This is serious—this is your health.

If modern medicine is so great, then why are we fatter and less healthy than ever? Why aren't we being educated on how to avoid the need for medications? Why isn't someone educating the patient about what they can do to reverse potentially serious problems by adjusting their diet, exercise, and exposure to toxins? When was the last time your doctor consulted with you about your diet? Has your doctor ever asked you what you eat and what your exercise habits are? Has your doctor advised you to limit certain foods like hydrogenated oils (read further about these fats in the nutrition chapter)? Hydrogenated oils cause heart disease; do you think that maybe your diet has any connection to your health? So many people never ask these questions, nor do they get advice on these issues. Why? Because if you lose, they lose! What you do get is a prescription that could potentially damage your health and cause unrelated problems. The only way to break out of this cycle is to repair your own health by making essential changes to your diet and lifestyle. Sometimes you will have to do this with the help of medication—know *your* options.

A major contributor to this problem is the fact that much of the medical student's curriculum focuses very little on nutrition and preventive medicine. Perhaps, what universities most need to do is alter their curriculum so that doctors can start to change more lives for the better.

I am not saying there has been a compromise of ethics by all doctors, but I hope I have your attention. I would like to point out that there are doctors who are aware of this ongoing epidemic, and are working to make changes. The Physicians Committee for Responsible Medicine, http://www. pcrm.org/, are doctors and laypersons working together for compassionate and effective medical practice, research, and health promotion. Maybe with their help, we can ensure that medical students get the proper nutrition training in medical school so that they emphasize prevention, especially prevention via diet. We need doctors to talk about how health is actually very simple! Eat a well-balanced, nutritional diet and limit processed foods. Make exercise a regular part of your life, including strength training and aerobic activity. I bet if you talked to the healthiest people you could find and asked them what prescription medications they are taking, chances are they will say *none*. Do not allow the drug companies to run your life—get that monkey off your back!

PART 2

Applications

Chapter Eight

Nutrition. Eat to Live, and Enjoy Yourself in the Process

"How we spend our days is, of course, how we spend our lives."
~Annie Dillard

"Forget past mistakes. Forget failures. Forget everything except what you're going to do now and do it."
~William Duran

"Nothing tastes as good as healthy feels."
~Unknown

The biggest and probably most difficult component of permanent weight loss is nutrition. For many of us, our monkey has complete control over our nutritional choices—either for emotional reasons or because of a lack of knowledge. This is when you have to ask yourself—are you eating out of boredom, depression, sadness, or happiness? Perhaps you think you are eating well. Why should someone be concerned with his or her eating? Nutritional, or dietary, factors contribute substantially to the burden of preventable illnesses and premature deaths in the United States.[1] A healthy, balanced diet provides the nutrition your body needs for energy and proper bodily functions. You need the appropriate fuel to keep your heart beating, your brain active, and your muscles working. Nutrients help build and strengthen bones, muscles, and tendons, and they regulate body processes such as blood pressure.

Due to the inconsistencies in the information available to them, most people do not know how to eat in a healthful manner. Consequently, many people jump from diet to diet, reaching out in the direction of the $30 billion dollar-per-year diet industry. Are you one of these people who are walking around in a fog?

Genetics, age, and gender are beyond your control, but you can manage your diet and master your metabolism.[2] You can lose weight through diet alone, but you can maximize weight loss and maintenance through diet *and* exercise. One pound of fat and one pound of muscle obviously weigh the same; however, because that one pound of muscle takes up less space and is active, it requires more calories even at rest. You *can* support and get the most out of your metabolic rate by adopting healthy eating and exercise habits.

I dedicated years to writing this book to help you reach the ultimate level of assurance and emotional power. The aim of this book was not to

1.   Frazao, E. The high costs of poor eating patterns in the United States. In: Frazao, E., ed. *America's Eating Habits: Changes and Consequences*. Washington, DC: U.S. Department of Agriculture (USDA), Economic Research Service (ERS), AIB-750, 1999.

2.   Sherry Holetzky, "*What is metabolism*," http://www.wisegeek.com/what-is-metabolism.htm, February 22, 2007.

give you a two-week diet, but rather to help you change your health and life permanently by assisting you to become the best you that you can be. During this journey, you will discover the positive attitude for which you have longed. Do not just read these pages without making the firm decision to act.

You must *believe* you can *succeed*. You *can* make it happen, if you *want* to make the changes—truly *want* to make the changes:

- Saying you want something is not enough. You must act on the words you tell yourself. If you want to be healthier, what steps are you taking to achieve that goal?

- Remember to **prioritize** and work on the issue that most needs changing (refer to Tables 1 and 3). Then work on the next when the first is under control.

- Be *sensible*—strive for *realistic* goals.

- Focus on what is *tangible*—bettering your health. Being healthier will create a more balanced and energetic you.

- Do not take the all-or-nothing approach and deprive yourself. You can have what you want in *moderation*, but you must take baby steps when embarking upon self-improvement projects.

- Allow each new modification to develop into a way of life before tackling the next.

Unlike many authors of diet books, I do not believe in eliminating foods, giving you a specific menu of items to eat, and then expecting your body and life to be different in two weeks' time. You are not really addressing your monkey by doing these things, and you will most likely revert to your old habits. I want you to learn sound, healthy eating habits. "Diet" typically implies that the nutritional changes you will be making are temporary. *There is nothing temporary about a healthy lifestyle.* Stop dieting and learn to make positive, permanent changes for life.

In order to achieve the pinnacle of health, be aware that your food choices deeply affect your vitality—poor food choices can cause an internal toxic overload.[3] We are eating out more and consuming more fast foods and more processed foods, which add little nutritional value to our diet. According to a 2000 study by the American Society for Clinical Nutrition, Americans are eating more meals outside the home, relying more heavily on convenience foods, and consuming larger food portions. In addition, according to the U.S. Department of Agriculture, Americans drank four times more milk than soda in 1945, and in 1998, they drank more than twice as much soda as milk. Is this true of your life?

I have spent a great deal of time studying the relationship between the foods people eat and their well-being, and in my opinion feel that many illnesses (previously mentioned) have a direct relation to our nutrition. I believe healthy changes in nutritional habits can decrease or possibly even eliminate many of these illnesses. Anyone who has personally witnessed these changes has come to the same conclusion. Talk to your doctor or internist and discover what you can do.

If you, like so many Americans, really are uncertain of what you should be eating, I recommend you hire a nutritionist or dietician; the investment would be worthwhile. By seeking out their help, you can create an eating lifestyle that you can maintain. Furthermore, countless books exist that can be of help. For example: the American Dietetic Association's *Complete Food and Nutrition Guide (Wiley;3 Rev upd edition September 18, 2006)* and *365 Days of Healthy Eating (Wiley)* can assist you in becoming educated on the subject of nutrition. Do not throw your money away on diet plans or pills that offer no bona fide long-term help; use the information I am providing, hire a nutritionist, or take the time to do your own research. You have already started by picking up this book! Educate yourself on reading food labels, understanding which foods pack the biggest nutritional punch, which foods you should always keep in your home, and which foods you never or rarely should keep in your home.

---

3. Dr. Paula Baillie-Hamilton, *Toxic Overload: A Doctor's Plan for Combating the Illnesses Caused by Chemicals in Our Foods, Our Homes, and Our Medicine Cabinets,* Part II The Chemical Connection to Chronic Illness, May 2005.

If you do not have Internet access and would like nutritional information, write to:

National Agricultural Library
Food and Nutrition Information Center
Nutrition.gov Staff
10301 Baltimore Avenue
Beltsville, MD 20705-2351

Some foods are just impossible to resist, and for that reason, we have a tendency to overindulge; therefore, I highly recommend you *not* keep these foods in your home. If the foods you give into most are not in your home, it will be easier to limit them to special occasions. I cannot keep sweets in my home; I love them, and I am very susceptible to them. I can polish off a bag of marshmallows, a pint of ice cream, a box of cookies—anything sweet—so I do *not* keep them in my home. Remember, you want to allow yourself treats, without being excessive.

I mentioned nutritional punch—by this, I mean a food's nutritional qualities. One calorie is a kilocalorie (kcal), which is the amount of energy required to raise one gram of water to one degree Celsius. According to this definition, all calories are equal. The effects of calories from different foods are what make calories different. What is the difference between 400 calories from chocolate ice cream and 400 calories from a blueberry, strawberry, and banana yogurt smoothie? You get calcium from the ice cream, which is good, but that is about it. From the smoothie, along with your 400 calories you get antioxidants, vitamins, calcium, and fiber. In addition, you can avoid saturated fat by using nonfat yogurt, compared to the high fat content of many brands of ice cream. Therefore, make choices that have healthful benefits.

Many overweight people complain that they cannot lose weight even though they do not eat very much. This is often true. However, in many cases, they are not eating big meals, yet the foods they do consume are calorie dense. All calories are effectively the same. The individual calories in a bowl of ice-cream are no more fattening than the individual calories in a comparable bowl of watermelon. The difference is that in equal volume, a bowl of ice cream has a greater number of calories than a bowl of watermelon; therefore, the ice cream *can* be more fattening. This is true because the ice cream contains more calories in equal proportion to the watermelon, not because they are different "types" of calories. In other words, foods differ significantly in the number of calories they contain in equal portions.

$$\frac{1}{2} \text{ cup vanilla ice cream} = 132 \text{ calories}$$
$$\frac{1}{2} \text{ cup (4 oz.) watermelon} = 54 \text{ calories}$$

You could eat 1 ½ cups of watermelon to equal a ½ cup of vanilla ice cream.

Therefore, portion size and nutritional quality are fundamental. Pay attention to the calories in a single serving size, because many small packaged foods will usually have multiple servings. We typically eat the whole package, thereby doubling or sometimes tripling our calories. You will be able to eat larger quantities of some foods, but you will have to limit your serving sizes of others.

Some of the science behind the calorie content of food is based on the fact that fat has nine calories for every gram, while carbohydrates and protein both have four calories for every gram. I encourage you to fill your diet with foods that are naturally lower in fat, such as whole grains, fruits, vegetables, and healthy fats (avocados, nuts, salmon, olive oil, etc.). Would you consider all calories equal? It is extremely important to understand that the total calories you consume each day will determine whether you gain, lose, or maintain weight. I encourage you to eat the foods that pack the best punch in a balanced manner.

Be aware that the junk foods most people love are typically much higher in calories and void of any nutrients. Not only are they high in calories but they have so many ingredients that I cannot even begin to pronounce, much less know what they are. Do you really want to be putting unidentified, unpronounceable crap in your body? Your body will not function to its optimal level on 1,800 calories of Twinkies. Instead, learn to balance and have fun with your diet. Longevity is the key, meaning that you must be able to support your diet decisions long-term. If you choose foods you enjoy, your eating plan will be one you can stick to, and that is one of the keys to successful weight loss.

In order to achieve overall nutritional success through weight loss or maintenance, we must become attuned with our bodies and their needs.

- **Assess your hunger.** Many people eat out of boredom, stress, because they have food in front of them, because they are distracted, or because the clock reads a certain time—not because they are truly hungry.

- **Master your internal cues.** Sit down at a table and eat slowly. Take the time to enjoy your food. Doing this will allow your brain the required time to relay the message of satisfaction to your stomach. *Eating should be enjoyable, not a race.*

- **Stop when you are satisfied, not when you are full.** Never stuff your face until you feel so full that you have to unbutton your pants. If you are no longer hungry and food remains on your plate, do not eat it; you can always save it for another day. Yes, it is OK to stop eating before you have finished everything on your plate; despite being told as a child that you must finish all of your food before being excused or before you are allowed dessert.

Sugar, is it metabolic poison?

As each diet enters into popularity, our numbness to food increases and the enjoyment it can truly bring decreases. The fact that the number of obese adults and children is spiraling out of control is a result of reduced activity, grotesque portions sizes, and consumption of high calorie foods. In my opinion, diets have been one of the catalysts to our obesity epidemic. We are relying on temporary dietary changes to fix an issue that requires permanent action.

I listed many of these temporary diets in the *Pardon Me While I Laugh* chapter. One of my favorites was the introduction of the low-fat diet craze in the 1980s and 1990s, which removed the fat from many of our favorite foods and replaced it with more sugar to compensate for loss of taste. While the food industry was trying to lower our overall fat intake, they did not lower our caloric intake. What exactly did they accomplish?

The food was lower in fat, but typically had the same amount of calories, if not more. Junk foods such as soft drinks, cakes, and cookies have high amounts of added sugar and squeeze healthier foods out of the diet. Remember that the bottom line in weight loss and maintenance boils down to calories *in* versus calories *out*. Without the proper guiding principles, people assumed that if the fat was gone, they could eat as much of these products as they pleased without consequence. However, the opposite happened, and people got fatter. Did this occur because sugar was bad? No, it was because people were dramatically increasing their calories *in* and did not manage their calories *out*. Just because something was lower in fat did not mean it was lower in calories. Ultimately, this diet did not fail anyone—people were just misinformed, and this is why I beg you to become educated. Do not make the same mistakes repeatedly.

Sugar continues to overrun our diet. Fruits contain simple sugars, but they also contain fiber, water, and vitamins, which make them a healthy choice. Snack foods, candy, and soda, on the other hand, often have large amounts of added sugars but little or no nutritional value. Most snack foods are high in sugar, providing "empty calories." These added sugars come in many different names (see the list below). Today's processed food is laden with sugar (see the list below). Without even knowing it, we have become a nation of excessive sugar consumers. Check the labels on the foods you eat, and see just how much added sugar you *are* getting.

Another reason you may be eating more sugar than you think is that some foods contain naturally occurring sugar, in addition to added sugars. The nutrition label does not break the sugars down separately by naturally occurring and added sugars. They are added together to give you one number. For example, 1 cup of plain, nonfat yogurt has 110 calories and 15 grams of sugar, while 1 cup of peach low-fat yogurt contains 220 calories and 38 grams of sugar. Lactose is the naturally occurring sugar in dairy products; therefore, by comparing these two products, you can see that the peach yogurt has approximately 23 grams of added sugar. Look at the ingredients in the product for added sugars.

Sugar, by any other name, is still sugar:

- Apple syrup
- Brown sugar
- Sugar (sucrose)
- Corn syrup
- Demerara
- Dextrose (glucose)
- Evaporated sugar cane juice
- Fructose
- Fruit juice concentrate
- High fructose corn syrup
- Honey
- Invert sugar
- Levulose (a technical name for fructose)
- Maltodextrin
- Maltose
- Maple syrup
- Molasses
- Muscovado or barbados
- Raw sugar
- Turbinado
- White grape juice concentrate

Most of my fond food memories are of sweets. The Good-Humor Man, birthdays with cake and ice cream, Halloween, holidays—you name it, and there were sweets piled high. I certainly am not complaining; I loved every minute of it. I would never suggest eliminating these foods, because I think sweets are wonderful! What I am suggesting is that you become aware of the sugar content in the foods you consume and manage the calories you are consuming.

Do not be hoodwinked by sugar marketing. Sugar is sugar, no matter how it might be packaged. Brown sugar and raw sugar are sucrose, just like white sugar; the only difference is that brown sugar and raw sugar may have had less processing than white sugar. Of course, it is better to avoid products that go through bleaching or exposing to chemicals; for that reason, I would suggest that you use raw sugar instead of white (bleached) sugar. The body typically uses sugar in any form in the same way, and sugar has the same caloric value no matter what the source. For you, a particular sugar will be unique for its taste and price. However, blackstrap molasses contains significant amounts of nutrients, such as manganese, copper, iron, calcium, potassium, magnesium, vitamin B6, and selenium.

While sugar itself is not going to make you fat, many of the foods eaten today are loaded with sugar, and as I have mentioned, the bottom line is calories *in* versus calories *out*. Therefore, anything with excess calories will make you gain weight. A teaspoon of sugar has 15 calories and 4 grams of carbohydrates. Carbohydrates provide energy, contain no fat, and like protein, contribute only four calories of energy in each gram (compared to the 9 calories in each gram of fat). In terms of total calories, refined sugars and natural sugars do not make a big difference. However, by increasing your consumption from natural sources such as fruits and grains, you also get other necessary nutrients not found in added sugars. Most added sugars do not contain vitamins or minerals; they are simply empty calories. For example, if you choose a 12 ounce soda loaded with 160 calories instead of 2 cups of blueberries with 180 calories, you will not benefit from the fiber, vitamins, and minerals that the blueberries contain. All fruits, vegetables, and dairy foods contain sugars; however, fruits, vegetables, and dairy products have nutrients that are helpful to the body, whereas added sugars such as white table sugar or high fructose corn syrup do not.

Supplementary sugars figure far too predominantly in our diets. Why do products such as peanut butter have added sugar, not to mention added fat? Our consumption of added sugars is on the rise. Lest we forget—more sugar means more calories. You can include sugars in your diet and still consume a healthful diet, but you must be smart about your overall caloric intake. Read the food labels! Sugar is not the "metabolic poison," as Robert Atkins calls it. Again, sugar alone does not make you fat; too many calories make you fat! Too much of anything will cause you to gain weight.

Here are some examples of foods with added sugar. Many of these foods are available sugar free. (Read the labels and make the right choice.)

- Applesauce
- Baked beans
- Barbeque sauce
- Breads
- Boxed macaroni and cheese
- Catsup
- Cereals
- Crackers
- Fruit juices—with added sugar
- Fruit yogurts
- Metamucil wafers (physillium husk fiber wafers)
- Pasta sauce
- Peanut butter
- Salad dressings
- Sodas

  The list goes on and on.

Please, take the time to look at the ingredients listed in your favorite foods and see where the added calories are hiding. How many different sugars are in one food, and how far up on the ingredients list are they? Educate yourself. There are options that have lower sugar or no sugar at all. The U.S. Department of Agriculture suggests keeping your sugar intake between 6 and 10 percent of your total calories; this is added sugar, not the naturally occurring sugar found in fruits, vegetables, or dairy products. Sugar itself does not pose any danger to our health; however, the food industry adds very large quantities of sugar, which causes us to consume an excess of calories. Excess calories make people fat, not sugar.

While I am guilty of replacing sugar with Splenda and other sugar substitutes (I too have some work to do), it is obviously not the key to weight loss. According to a national survey by the Calorie Control Council, by 2004, 180 million Americans were buying sugar-free products, up from 109 million in 1991. A 2005 report by A.C. Nielsen found that while the low-carb craze was fading, low-sugar packaged items represented the second-fastest-growing division (behind organics) in the good-for-you product industry. In addition, while these products have increased in sales, our waistlines have continued to grow. A teaspoon of raw sugar in your coffee will not kill you, and if you really want something sweet—eat it, but in moderation. You can have your cake and eat it too—but in *moderation*!

In other words, leave the Twinkies and ice cream for infrequent occasions, and start eating the nutrient-dense foods that will keep you satisfied between meals, make you feel more energized, and have health benefits. For example, berries such as blueberries, raspberries, and strawberries, and vegetables such as tomatoes, spinach, squash, sweet potatoes, and carrots, are all high in vitamins, antioxidants, and fiber. Even though oxygen is an essential element of life, it also creates damaging by-products known as free radicals.[4] Free radicals are the result of many environmental pollutants. Some believe that in animal tissues, free radicals can damage cells and accelerate the progression of cancer, cardiovascular disease, and age-related diseases. Free radicals can cause numerous problems, including heart damage and a weakening of the immune system. Antioxidant rich foods will help defend your body

---

4.   http://ask.yahoo.com/20020926.html, Definition: Free Radical, *Britannica Concise*, February 6, 2007.

against these "trespassers." Antioxidants act as cell protectors and neutralize free radicals by helping to prevent cell and tissue damage. Antioxidants come in a variety of forms and include, but are not limited to, vitamins A, C, and E, carotenoids, and selenium. You will find the highest concentrations in the most deeply or brightly colored fruits and vegetables. Many people try to get their antioxidants through supplements and recent findings published in the Journal of the American Medical Association study suggest people get their antioxidants and vitamins through foods, not supplementation.[5] Remember: while Twinkies and french fries taste great, they are not providing any health benefits.

---

5.   Rob Stein, "Antioxidant Supplements Don't Extend Life Span, Study Finds," *The Washington Post*, February 28, 2007; A06.

> **So what happens to the calories you eat:**

As you make adjustments to your eating, understand that regardless of where your calories come from, your body converts your calories into physical energy or stores them within your body as fat. There are three ways to keep these calories from being stored as fat: one, by reducing the calories you consume; two, by increasing your physical activity to burn more calories; and three, combining both calorie reduction and physical activity. Simple enough, right?

3,500 calories = 1 pound
To lose 1 pound (of fat), you must subtract 3,500 calories

Options:
Subtract 3,500 calories from your diet
(subtract 500 calories a day from your diet: 500 calories x 7 days a week = 3,500 calories a week)

Or
Burn 3,500 calories through movement
(burn 500 calories a day through exercise: 500 calories x 7 days a week = 3,500 calories a week)

Or
You can lose 1 pound through a combination of diet and exercise
(cut 250 calories a day from your diet and burn 250 calories a day through exercise)
(cut 300 calories a day from your diet and 200 calories a day through exercise)
(find the balance that is right for you)
(500 calories x 7 days a week = 3,500 calories a week)

➤ **As you drop weight, your caloric needs will change.** What you needed at 200 pounds will be less than what you needs at 175 pounds, and so on. So, make sure that as you make progress on your road to well-being, you manage your caloric intake accordingly. Many Web sites can be helpful in determining the calories you will need for weight loss and maintenance based on your age, height, current weight, and activity level. I like the site www.caloriecontrol.org.

When making changes to your diet, be sure to include your favorite foods. You do not have to eliminate the foods you love; you just have to learn to make smarter choices. If you are someone like me who likes to have dessert after dinner, just make it a healthier dessert. For example, if you normally eat a pint of ice cream, substitute a fudge bar, frozen fruit bar, frozen grapes, or plain fruit. You can freeze yogurt with added fruit and honey and have that for dessert. The healthier options are endless. *Lifestyle changes are not about going cold turkey or turning your life upside down; instead, they are about learning to make healthier replacements for your current choices.* Nevertheless, making improved substitutions does not mean you can eat as much as you want; you can still gain weight eating healthily if you are consuming too many calories. Remember, weight loss, gain, or maintenance is about "calories *in* versus calories *out*."

Your diet history, eating habits, and lifestyle will all have an effect on your new nutritional goals. You must customize your individual food preferences. For healthier cooking, you can find great light recipes at www.cookinglight.com, www.epicurious.com, and www.foodnetwork.com.

Now is the time to change your life! The road to change:

★ Remember to prioritize; do not try to work on everything at once.

1. **Assess your daily eating habits.** Incorporate healthy eating as a way of life. These changes must be practical and maintainable. Pay attention to your hunger cues! Remember to make prioritized changes such as taking control of your environment—see No. 8.

2. **Start your day off right by having a well-balanced breakfast.** Your body receives no food (fuel) between your last meal of one day and your first meal of the next. Breakfast is essential to jump-starting your engine. Just as you cannot run your car without gas, you cannot run the body without fuel. If the cells in the body do not receive the nutrients they need to function, they will store fat to compensate for times of deprivation. Consequently, if you skip breakfast, you skip the opportunity to put your metabolism into high gear. You have hundreds of choices for breakfast—make smart ones. See **Table 6** for a list of a few of the endless options.

3. **Do not skip meals.** Many times people will skip a meal so that they can save calories for later. Unfortunately, while this looks good on paper, we usually wind up binging because we are ravenous. Eat lighter meals if you plan to indulge, but do not forgo a meal altogether.

4. **Eat balanced meals.** The body needs a constant supply (small servings) of nutrients to perform efficiently. This includes a balance of carbohydrates, proteins, and fats. Try to limit processed foods and refined sugars. Moderation is the key.

5. **Variety is good and helps keep you focused and happy.** You can improvise and find what you like. Remember to use natural foods and lower fat options where and when available. For easy meals, get a Crock-Pot, a grill, a wok, or even a steamer to start cooking better. These Web sites can help with new recipes so you don't become

stuck for ideas: www.cookinglight.com, www.epicurious.com, and www.foodnetwork.com.

6. **Eat small meals often** (not for everyone). Do you ever go too long without eating and find yourself eating everything and anything in sight? Eating smaller, more frequent meals helps eliminate this scenario by stabilizing blood sugar, keeping your metabolism fully charged, and assisting the body in maintaining a constant state of efficiency. When sugar levels drop, you become exceedingly hungry and will tend to overeat. Your blood sugar drops at regular intervals throughout the day. Usually, you can feel the drop in the form of sluggishness or mental exhaustion. Your brain realizes the need for energy and sends an SOS through the nervous system saying, "Feed me." One part of the message causes your stomach to growl. You need to identify the early stages of hunger so that you do not wait until you are completely on empty before refueling. That is why I encourage eating smaller meals throughout the day, so that you never let the blood sugar levels get too low and cause severe overeating. If you tend to overeat with this method, I suggest you stick to three balanced meals a day.

7. **Eat slowly and *stop* when you are *satisfied*, not stuffed.** It takes time for the brain to realize that the stomach is full, so do not eat too quickly. Slow down and enjoy your food. Take the time to enjoy what you are eating. Be aware of your eating, and stop when you are satisfied, not stuffed. Only you can make the changes necessary to improve your life. These changes will be worth it in the end. Eating more slowly will allow the brain to register that it is satisfied; for that reason, be aware of what and how quickly you are eating.

8. **Take charge of your environment!** After you have served yourself a reasonable plate of food, put the rest away, sit down, and eat. Do not sit in front of the TV, where you will eat mindlessly. Eat at the table. Enjoy what you have prepared, and take the time to feel your body getting satisfied. *Please, eliminate the distractions.* By having put the rest of the food away, you will have to make a conscious effort to have seconds. Moreover, by sitting down without the TV,

you allow yourself to focus entirely on the meal, and thus you will be aware of your satisfaction point. In fact, once you learn to identify the point where your body is satisfied, you will no longer want to overeat. The truth is eating just the right amount feels a lot better than feeling "full." You will find if you do not deprive yourself and pay attention to what you are doing, you will usually not overeat. Sometimes it is impossible to sit down and eat your meals, but be cognizant of the fact that most people who eat on the run tend to eat convenient foods loaded with fat and calories. We tend to eat most "convenient" foods (fast foods) too quickly, which leads to overeating because we are not allowing the brain adequate time to signal it has had enough. Take control of your environment!

9. **It's OK to have treats.** If you allow yourself a piece of cake, chocolate, or an alcoholic beverage, enjoy it—do not feel guilty and throw in the towel. It is OK to enjoy yourself—in moderation.

10. **Manage cravings and overeating:**

    a. If you really want something, do not deny yourself the pleasure. Denying yourself can result in overindulging. You have the ability to say when and how much. This is about choice and control—you have both! A craving is typically satisfied within the first three bites.

    b. Do not go grocery shopping when you are hungry, because it will trigger binges.

    c. Follow #8.

11. **Do not exclude your favorite foods.** If you cannot resist overindulging on a particular food (for me, that would be anything sweet), do not keep it in your house. This will force you to have to go out and get it as a single serving. I love ice cream for dessert, but I have no control over sweets; therefore, instead of sabotaging myself, I take a walk to the soft serve yogurt place about one mile from my house to get my "fix." I eat my yogurt, guilt free, as I walk back home. You see, not only did I get some exercise after dinner, but I also enjoyed dessert and felt good about it. I do this about five

times a week. I ate my monkey; now you too must get your monkey off your back.

12. **Keep healthful foods in the house and keep them as conveniently located as possible.** If that requires cutting up fruit or vegetables on Sunday for the week to come, do it. You can also plan your menu over the weekend for the week to come. I sometimes cook big portions of things and freeze what I am not going to eat that night. When I have a tight schedule, I can simply grab something I made out of the freezer and heat it up. This works for just about anything, from my delicious vegetarian chili to my vegetarian lasagna. Meals and snacks do not have to be challenging. Furthermore, remember to spice up your foods to give them flavor and variety. If your food tastes good, you will enjoy eating healthy.

13. **Start a *food journal* in order to stay the course of your *nutritional goals.*** Set realistic, quantifiable goals and stick to them. People who monitor their food intake lose more weight than those who do not. A food journal can be the key to both short-term and long-term weight loss, because recording everything you eat helps you see what, how much, when, and why you are eating. Include every thing—even a little bite of something (butter on your bagel oᵗ handful of popcorn at the movies). Many people notice that t᾿ eat considerably more than they had thought because the ni' make a material difference in caloric intake. Writing down thing you consume makes you further accountable to yourᵗ discourages mindless eating. The journal can help you fi where you can and need to make adjustments. When writᵗ it is very hard to be in denial about poor eating habits with yourself! See Table 7.

14. **Make healthier substitutions.** It can be as easy as usᵗ low-fat milk in your coffee instead of cream, hᵢ whole milk, or ordering a fat-free drink from youᵤ shop instead of one with whole milk. If you elimᵢ cream, you will save even more calories. Let the a treat that you have once a week, or once a ᴍ

your habits. Changing your condiments can help you save hundreds of calories. For example, instead of using mayonnaise, switch to dijonnaise or spicy mustard. You can convert most recipes to be low-fat, low-sugar, and low-sodium. There are plenty of options to help you lower calories and fat. The small changes have the biggest impact without causing major overhauls. See **Tables 8 and 8A.**

15. **Learn to be a smart shopper.** Learning more about food labels is an important step you cannot skip on your way to nutritional education:

   a. **Serving Size:** The Food and Drug Administration says that a single serving size measurement is a reflection of what people actually consume. This is rarely the case. Most people do not stop at one serving; they eat three or four servings and seldom consider the increased caloric intake. Therefore, if there are two servings in the package and you eat the entire package, you must double all of the nutritional information listed. Also, be aware that serving sizes are not uniform: a box of raisin bran can have 200 calories for a *half cup* serving, while a box of puffed rice cereal can have 220 calories for a *one cup* serving; therefore, the raisin bran is higher in calories in proportion to the puffed rice. If you eat cereal, measure the amount after you have served yourself and see how many servings you are truly eating. Be aware of what in reality is one serving.

   b. **Fats:** Be sure to know what types of fats are in the foods you eat. The label will list saturated fats (artery clogging fats) and unsaturated fats (monounsaturated and polyunsaturated, the "healthier fats" that help to lower LDL, or bad cholesterol). For example, olive oil, canola oil, and avocados are high in monounsaturated fat, while sunflower oil, corn oil and most seeds and nuts are high in polyunsaturated fat. It is important to include these healthier fats in your daily eating—in moderation. Try to reduce your consumption of saturated fats. Most saturated fats come from animal products, whole milk dairy products, and some plants such as coconuts. In addition, try to limit your consumption of the unhealthy fat called trans fat. Trans fats are *added* to many of the foods that people enjoy on a daily basis. Trans fats are used to increase shelf life, taste, and crunch. These fats are usually on the ingredient label as partially hydrogenated or hydrogenated oils. You will find trans fat in microwave popcorn, chips, dips, non-dairy whipped topping, margarine, candies, etc. The list goes on and on, and I will talk about this fat again toward the end of this chapter. Healthcare organizations recommend we limit our fat (any type) consumption to 30 percent of our total caloric intake. For more on trans fats, read the trans fat section below.

c. **Fiber:** Fiber is an important component of your healthy diet, and the recommended daily allowance of fiber is between 25 and 35 grams. Fiber offers exercise for your intestines—a workout for the colon, if you will. Soluble fiber can reduce cholesterol levels and thereby decrease the risk of heart disease. Along with a low-fat diet, a high fiber intake could help reduce the risk of certain cancers, including colon and rectal cancer. Add fiber into the diet slowly to avoid bloat and discomfort. If you just cannot let go of a lower fiber cereal, blend it with some higher fiber cereal. The best sources of fiber are oats, barley, brown rice, beans (lentil, black-eyed peas, black beans, chickpeas, etc.), kasha (buckwheat), fruits (dried figs, apples with the skin, raspberries, etc.) and vegetables (peas, cooked spinach, yams with the skin, etc.). Fiber fills you up and helps keep you satisfied longer.

d. **Proteins:** Proteins are essential for growth and repair. They play a crucial role in virtually all biological processes in the body such as muscle contraction, immune protection, and the transmission of nerve impulses. The Recommended Daily Allowance (RDA) of protein according to U.S. government standards is 0.8 gram per 2.2 pounds of *ideal* body weight for an adult. The RDA says this amount of protein meets 97.5 percent of the population's needs. With the high protein diet craze, we have lost sight of how much protein we should be eating. There are numerous quality sources of protein from which to choose. I suggest fish, low-fat dairy products, eggs, legumes, and soy products (tofu, soymilk, etc.). If you eat meat, please find lean, hormone-free cuts.

e. **Sodium:** The RDA (Recommended Dietary Allowance) of sodium is 2,400 milligrams per day. Remember that this includes table salt as well as salt that is already in foods. On average, we consume 2,500–5,000 milligrams a day, entirely too much. There is a link to high sodium intake and high blood pressure. Learn to read the label and pay attention to the sodium content and serving size. Look for labels that say low in sodium, salt-free or unsalted. Be sure to look closely at processed foods, canned foods, and packaged meats; all are characteristically high in sodium.

f. **Ingredients:** Can you recognize the ingredients in the foods you eat? I have a rule of thumb—if I cannot pronounce it, I do not eat it. Look for natural foods that are as close to their original form as possible. Stay away from preservatives and fillers that you cannot pronounce. Foods are best in their most natural state.

g. **Order of the ingredients:** Ingredients listed are in order by weight, from the greatest to the least. Choose items that tend to have shorter lists with natural, healthy ingredients first.

That Special Problem: Eating Out

Fast Food

If fast food is your only option, make an effort to choose the healthier items on the menu. If fast food places listed the calories next to each menu item, would you reconsider your choice? An FYI: the most health-conscience consumers eat out the least.

Here are some options for you when you visit your local fast food places. These are approximate calories:

Arby's

Grilled Chicken Deluxe	**295 calories**

(skip the honey mustard sauce, instead use ½ a packet of the Arby's sauce)

Regular Roast Beef	350 calories
Big Montana Roast Beef Sandwich	630 calories

- o   To find out more about Arby's menu, visit http://www.arbysrestaurants.com/

Burger King

BK Veggie Burger w/ reduced fat mayo	**340 calories**
Grilled Chicken Whopper Jr. no mayo	**350 calories**
Original Chicken Whopper	580 calories (26 grams of fat)
Original Whopper Jr., without mayo	310 calories
Original Whopper with cheese	800 calories
Double Whopper	980 calories
BK Stacker	1,000 calories (68 grams of fat)

- o   Find all of Burger King's nutritional information at http://www.bk.com/Food/Nutrition/index.aspx

Kentucky Fried Chicken

Original Chicken Breast no skin or breading	**180 calories**
Tender Roast Sandwich without sauce	318 calories
Large Popcorn Chicken	660 calories
Extra Crispy plus Original Recipe thigh	820 calories

- o   All of the menu items and their nutritional values can be found at www.yum.com/nutrition/menu.asp?brandID_Abbr=2_KFC

McDonald's

Fruit n' Yogurt Parfait without granola	130 calories
Fruit n' Yogurt Parfait with granola	160 calories
McGrilled Chicken without mayo	340 calories
McGrilled Chicken with mayo	400 calories
Crispy Chicken	500 calories
McDonald's Go Active Happy Meal w/out the dressing	270 calories
w/ low fat balsamic vinaigrette	310 calories
w/regular dressing	560 calories
Regular Hamburger	260 calories
Hamburger with cheese	310 calories
Double Cheeseburger	460 calories
Big-Mac	560 calories
The Chocolate Triple Thick Shake, 32 oz.	1160 calories

Which of these do you think would be the smartest choice?

Egg McMuffin	**290 calories**
Sausage McMuffin	370 calories
Bacon, Egg and Cheese Biscuit	440 calories
Sausage Biscuit with Egg	500 calories
Egg and Cheese McGriddle	560 calories
Spanish Omelet Bagel	710 calories
Big Breakfast	730 calories
Deluxe Breakfast	1,220 calories

o All of these items and their caloric values came straight off their Web site at www.mcdonalds.com

Pizza Hut

Fit n' Delicious Pizza, two slices w/vegetable toppings	**280-300 calories**
Thin n' Crispy-Veggie Lover's, two slices	**340-360 calories**

✓ Stay away from stuffed crusts and meat lovers. Too much of everything = far too many calories.

o Visit http://www.pizzahut.com for their nutritional values and some helpful tips to eating better and living better.

Subway

All are 6", on white or wheat with lettuce, tomatoes, pickles, onions, and olives without any added condiments.

Veggie Delite	230 calories
Roast Beef	290 calories
Honey Mustard Ham	320 calories
Oven Roasted Chicken	330 calories

✓ Stay away from the Meatball marinara, Tuna (made with tons of mayonnaise), Pastrami, and Spicy Italian.

Also, be aware of the condiments you add. You will have to add them to the total calories of your sandwiches:

2 Tbsp. spicy mustard	5 calories
1 Tbsp. light mayo	45 calories
1 Tbsp. chipotle sauce	100 calories
1 Tbsp. mayo	110 calories

o All of the nutritional information for Subway can be gathered at www.subway.com

Taco Bell

Grilled Chicken or Steak Soft tacos Fresco Style (2)	340 calories
Bean Burrito, Fresco style	350 calories

✓ Taco Bell designed their Fresco Style menu to be lower in fat.

✓ Stay away from Grilled Stuffed Burritos, Nachos Bell-Grandes, and Quesadillas, and most of their specialty items.

o You can find all of Taco Bell's nutritional information at www.taco-bell. com/nutrition.htm.

➢ **Most fast food restaurants will have these guides available for you—take advantage of them.** The more you know, the better off you will be. For those of you that will be making road trips, you can now make informed decisions about what you are going to eat.

Restaurants:

One of my biggest pet peeves is the all-you-can-eat buffet. Why would you ever go to an all-you-can-eat buffet? Have you ever heard the phrase, you are what you eat? All-you-can-eat restaurants will make losing weight impossible. *I* cannot control myself in all-you-can-eat restaurants, and I cannot imagine that most people can. Take control and make smart choices when going to your favorite restaurants.

Restaurant meals are definitely tasty and convenient, but they are not always great for your waistline. People who eat out often are people who consume more calories. You do not have control of ingredients and portion size. As I have said, usually if it is in front of you, you will eat it, and all of it.

Know how it is cooked or prepared. Try to minimize your consumption of these preparations:
- Aioli (garlic-flavored oil or mayonnaise)
- Alfredo (butter, cream, or cheese base)
- Alla crema (a cream sauce)
- Au beurre (with butter)
- Au gratin (topped with cheese and buttered breadcrumbs)
- Breaded
- Battered
- Crispy (usually means fried)
- Deep fried
- Fritto (fried)
- Graisse (fat or grease)
- Pan-fried

Instead, try:
- Alla griglia (grilled)
- Au jus (pan juices)
- Au natural (plainly cooked)

- Baked
- Blackened
- Blanched (quickly plunged into boiling water)
- Boiled
- Broiled or charbroiled
- Grilled

Some conscious food decisions that will help you gain control:

- Ask your server to remove from the table or not bring the breadbasket
- Ask your server to remove from the table or not bring the chips and salsa
- Replace your salad dressing with olive oil and vinegar
- If you do eat bread, dip it in olive oil instead of using butter
- Eat skinless, white meat chicken
- Have a salad (dressing on the side, lemon, or olive oil and vinegar) or broth-based soup instead of an appetizer
- Eat Canadian bacon instead of sausage
- Order a roasted vegetable pizza with a whole-wheat crust, and ask for light or no cheese
- Order your sauces and salad dressings on the side so you can control how much you use
- Stick to the leanest cuts of meat (buffalo, round, sirloin, filet minion, and flank) and eat free-range or organic when possible
- Watch out for cream-based soups (chowders, bisques); instead have a broth-based soup

Ask questions so that you understand how your food is prepared. Tell your server that you are trying to eat healthily and ask what the healthiest selections are. Most restaurants understand the growing demand for healthy alternatives.

If everyone else has dessert, you can too—just remember there are some healthier alternatives. Most places will have sorbets or fresh fruit. If you want a truly rich dessert, try to split it with someone, or ask your server for half an order. You do not have to miss all the fun; however, you cannot eat heavy foods all the time and expect to see changes in your waistline or health. Make smart choices that support your overall health goals.

If you are on a long road trip, plan to stop for healthy meals. In the nutrition section of this book, I talk about most restaurants having their menus available on-line with their full nutritional values. Before a trip, take the time to research which places are the best to stop and what to eat there. Also, there are many books on the market that are specifically for dining out, so you can always have a guide like that as well.

However, since you do not have 100 percent control over how your meals are prepared when you dine out, save restaurants for special occasions. When eating at home, *have fun with your shopping and try new things.* You will be amazed at how much more you will enjoy your food and how much better you will feel. Cook your meals from fresh ingredients and avoid premade foods. Many prepackaged foods contain ingredients you cannot pronounce, such as EDTA (ethylenediamine tetra acetic acid), ascorbic acid, sulfites, dextrose, guar gum, Carrageenan, and yellow no. 5, just to name a few. I didn't even know what most of them were until I did some research. Most of these items are preservatives that allow your foods a longer shelf life. Look at what is in your pantry, and if the labels read a lot like those in your medicine cabinet, you should make some adjustments.

Trans Fats/ Trans Fatty Acids

Trans fatty acids are "additives" that I encourage you to remove from your diet because they are difficult to digest, have the potential to raise bad cholesterol, and can dramatically increase your risk for heart disease. Trans fats are unnecessary in healthful foods. These fats have made cookies, potato chips, and crackers crispier and cheaper to make, and by filling their fryers with it, restaurants enjoy longer fryer life at lower cost. Since trans fats turn solid at room temperature, manufacturers can infuse foods with them, thus creating the junk food world as we know it. The FDA estimates that 42,000 products contain partially hydrogenated oils as one of their primary ingredients. Look for the words "hydrogenated" or "partially hydrogenated" in the ingredients of the foods in your home. There are several companies that make "trans-fat free" products so you can still enjoy some of your favorite snacks.

The FDA has been paying attention to this fat, and I'm sure that the edible-oil industries are terrified of us finding out about all their terrible fats and are creating as many roadblocks as possible. Remember, the tobacco industry was diligent in covering up the harmful effects of cigarettes for decades, and when uncovered, people kept smoking. I, for one, want to know what I am eating. Do you?

Be careful—products can be cholesterol-free and saturated-fat-free and still have trans fats. Become aware of which products you should make scarce. Limit the amount of processed and fast foods that you eat, especially fried fast foods. Be careful, because some companies have eliminated trans fats by substituting palm and coconut kernel oils, which happen to be the worst of the saturated fats.

Be aware of these foods:
- Non-dairy creamers
- Margarine
- Microwave popcorn
- Chips
- Cookies such as Nabisco Chips Ahoy
- Granola Bars
- Krispy Kremes
- Many boxed cereals such as Cracklin' Oat Bran, Cocoa Pebbles, etc.
- Crackers such as Wheat Thins and Keebler Club
- Canned foods such as Campbell's Chunky Sirloin Burger

Many companies are hearing our cries and making changes. Kraft and Frito-Lay are two companies removing trans fats or at least providing other options; however, the only way to eliminate most additives from your diet is to avoid foods that contain them and instead eat as much fresh, unprocessed food as possible. You will feel the difference, because your body will not have to work overtime to digest these chemical additions. The main function of your digestive system is to digest food, not breakdown foreign substances. There are already enough pollutants in the air for your body to filter—do not give it additional work. Is it any wonder we are sick and lethargic?

Table 5:
Recap: some of the tools to *get that monkey off your back.*

1. **Assess your daily eating habits with the help of a food journal:**
   - ✓ Specify your eating and exercise goals—prioritize, do not try to do everything at once
   - ✓ Are you truly hungry
   - ✓ Include everything, even the smallest bite of something
   - ✓ Gain knowledge of your eating habits

2. **Eat balanced meals, starting with breakfast:**
   - ✓ Start the day off right with an energy-packed breakfast
   - ✓ Make smart choices from every food group
   - ✓ Get the most nutrition out of your calories
   - ✓ Eat as many natural foods as possible

3. **Variety is good:**
   - ✓ Use spices
   - ✓ Try different recipes regularly

4. **Eat smaller meals often to prevent overeating:**
   - ✓ Keep your body in a constant state of efficiency
   - ✓ Maintain blood sugar levels to avoid overeating

5. **Slow down and enjoy your food:**
   - ✓ Take the time and chew your food slowly
   - ✓ Enjoy what you're eating
   - ✓ Allow your brain to process the act of eating and allow it to register satiety
   - ✓ Stop before you're stuffed

6. **Take charge of your environment:**
   - ✓ Serve yourself and others once and then put the food away
   - ✓ Sit without distractions—no TV

✓ Focus on your food and when you become satisfied

7. **Do not exclude your favorite foods:**
   ✓ Try lighter versions of your favorite foods
   ✓ Enjoy treats in moderation

8. **Keep healthy foods accessible:**
   ✓ Keep fruits in a bowl, on the counter, or on the top shelf in the fridge
   ✓ Keep vegetables where you can see them and grab quickly

9. **Make healthy substitutions:**
   ✓ The smallest modifications generate the biggest rewards
   ✓ It can be as simple as switching from whole milk to fat-free or low-fat milk

10. **Learn to be a smart shopper:**
    ✓ Read labels: know what one serving size is; know the ingredients
    ✓ Fill your basket or cart with healthful items

➢ Very helpful tools:
www.mypyramid.gov
www.nal.usda.gov/fnic/
www.nutrition.org/

Remember

- Caloric Intake > Calories Used = *Weight Gain*
- Caloric Intake < Calories Used = *Weight Loss*
- Caloric Intake = Calories Used = *Weight Control*

  ➢ **Please note:** If you are pregnant or wish to become pregnant, pregnancy is not an excuse to consume all-you-can-eat. The general recommendation is that a pregnant women increase her food by 100 calories during the first trimester and 300 calories in the second and third trimester. Four marshmallows are the equivalent of 100 calories, so mind the binges. Talk with your OBGYN.

Make the commitment to eat for a new and improved you. One of your goals will be to consume as much nutrition as possible while maintaining a reasonable number of calories and enjoying yourself without obsessing over each bite you take—get that monkey off your back!

Table 6:

Start your day off right by having a well-balanced breakfast.

a. Oatmeal made with fat-free or low-fat milk and raisins and a piece of fruit

b. A fruit smoothie made with plain fat-free or low-fat yogurt, blueberries, pineapple, banana, and mango (you can use any combination of fruit) with a piece of toast

c. Fat-free or low-fat cottage cheese with wheat germ and molasses and a bunch of grapes

d. Bran (or another high fiber cereal) with fat-free or low-fat milk and a piece of fruit

e. Oatmeal pancakes with real maple syrup and fresh fruit

f. Four egg whites and one whole egg or egg substitute scrambled with vegetables and fat-free or low-fat cheese, a piece of whole-wheat toast, and a piece of fruit

g. One egg mixed with fat-free or low-fat milk (to add volume) and fat-free or low-fat cottage cheese, a piece of fruit, and a piece of toast

h. Fat-free or low-fat yogurt with low fat granola and berries (blueberries, raspberries, blackberries, etc.)

i. Whole grain toast with natural peanut butter, a piece of fruit, and a small glass of fat-free or low-fat milk

j. An egg white omelet with fat-free or low-fat ricotta cheese and fresh basil, a piece of whole grain toast, and a piece of fruit or a glass of full-pulp juice—I prefer to do egg whites with one egg yolk (three eggs total)

k. Half a melon filled with fat-free or low-fat yogurt and blueberries or any other fruit

l. Whole wheat English muffin with natural peanut butter and a cup of fat-free or low-fat yogurt with blueberries

m. Whole wheat English muffin topped with egg whites mixed with two tablespoons of fat-free or low-fat cottage cheese and fruit such as papaya, mango, pineapple, apple, etc.

n. Filling options for omelets: artichoke, tomato, spinach, broccoli, zucchini, mushrooms, onions, healthy homemade chili (vegetarian), low-fat cottage cheese, light cheese, etc.

o. Pair your omelet with a fresh-squeezed juice or a fresh piece of fruit

Table 7:
Write it down. Food Journal.

a. **What:** What you ate, specifically—even if it was one bite of a pizza or three tortilla chips.

b. **How much:** Did you eat one serving of cereal, or was it four? Be specific—saying one bowl of cereal does not accurately convey the amount! If you need to measure your food in order to gauge your serving sizes, I encourage you to do so.

c. **When:** The time you consumed each meal, snack, or nibble.

d. **Where:** Where you were when you consumed each meal, snack, or nibble.

e. **Feelings:** Recording how you feel after you eat can help uncover patterns to emotional eating (try to do this within fifteen minutes of eating). I found that when I was home with nothing much to do, I ate purely out of boredom. Uncovering this behavioral pattern led me to make a change. Now, I keep myself active with other things and try to eliminate the mindless snacking. I have also eliminated my easy-to-go-to foods like chips and salsa and replaced them with crunchy vegetables in the event that a nibble need arises. When I feel completely overwhelmed by food, I go for a walk. Incorporate these changes gradually; otherwise, it will be very frustrating.

f. **How many calories did you consume:** Add up your calories and see how much you are have truly eaten.

g. **At the end of the first week, determine if there is a need to make a change:** Write down your intention to make a change. Take this change and apply it to the following week. Is this change reasonable? Is this change sustainable?

h. **Review your journal (read aloud) monthly:** Determine patterns, weaknesses, emotional connections, etc. Was your one change effective—why or why not? Do you need to make a different change? Stick with your change until it becomes second nature then make a new change.

Table 8:

What changes can you make?

You can choose lighter versions of food items and save calories without much sacrifice. Remember that liquids have calories as well, unless it is just plain old water. These are the average calories of each item:

Beer, 12 oz.	
Light	*99*
Regular	146
Wine, 3.5 fl. oz	
White	*70*
Red	74
Mixed drinks, 6 oz.	
Bloody Mary	*138*
Daiquiri	333
Pina Colada	325
Soda pop, 12 fl. oz	
Diet	*4*
Regular	152

Simple substitutions that can and will make a difference:

Cream cheese, 1 Tbsp.	
Fat-free	*15*
Light	35
Regular	51
Ricotta, 1 cup	
Part skim	*340*
Whole	428

Sour Cream, 1 Tbsp.
Fat-Free	*12*
Light	20
Regular	26

Ice cream versus frozen yogurt, chocolate ½ cup
Yogurt	*115*
Ice cream	143

Milk, 1 cup
Skim/Fat-Free	*86*
1%	102
2%	121
Whole	150

Mayonnaise, 1 Tbsp.
Fat-free	*10*
Light	49
Regular	99

Salad Dressings, 1 Tbsp.
Blue Cheese
Low Cal	*25*
Regular	77

French
Low cal	*22*
Regular	67

Italian
Low Cal	*16*
Regular	69
Olive Oil and Vinegar	*70*

Tuna, 3 oz. chunk light
    Water packed   *99*
    Oil packed   168

Popcorn, 1 cup
    Air popped   *31*
    Oil popped   55

Pie, 1/6 of an 8"
    Pumpkin   *229*
    Apple   277
    Chocolate   344
    Pecan   452

Tortillas, 6"
    Corn   *58*
    Flour   104

Breakfast
    English muffin with egg, cheese, and Canadian bacon   *289*
    Croissant with egg and sausage   413
    Biscuit with egg and sausage   581

French fries
    Small   *291*
    Medium   458
    Large   578

Hamburger, 1
    Single patty   *272*
    Double patty   576

As you can see, there are small changes that will make a healthier lifestyle very easy. You will be surprised at the difference these small adjustments can make. *Pick the lower calorie versions whenever possible.*

Table 8A:
Small changes that make a huge impact without sacrificing flavor.

- Choose baked, broiled, or grilled over fried
- Choose low-fat options over their full fat counterparts (but be aware of increased sugar content)
- Skip the mayo and opt for mustard or dijonnaise
- Cook with nonfat spray to eliminate calories
- Eat child-size portions
- Skip the cheese or opt for light or fat-free cheese
- Order salad dressing on the side, and use your fork to dip in the dressing
- Order an appetizer instead of a main dish
- If you eat red meat, select leaner cuts like sirloin steak or filet mignon, or pot roast instead of hamburgers or meat loaf
- Chose grilled or baked seafood over fried seafood dishes
- Share a main course
  - ➤ **You can find nutritional information for any food item at** http://www.nal.usda.gov/fnic/foodcomp/search/

Chapter Nine

Exercise! For a Healthy Heart and Lungs! Burn Calories and Fat! Lower Stress and *Boost* Your Energy! Go Ahead and Sweat! And Have Better *Sex!*

"There is no shortcut to winning and success. There is only getting started and sticking to it."
~Anonymous

"The journey is not hard. It only seems hard because the human mind fears the river and avoids the mountain."
~Author Unknown

"Everything is possible; it's just that the impossible things take a little longer to figure out!"
~Author Unknown

I hope that I have brought some clarity to the confusing matter of nutrition, so let me get into the importance of exercise. Exercise does not have to be confusing. The television, radio, magazines, and even the Internet inundated us with information on how to exercise, when to exercise, and how long to exercise. You do not have to bend yourself in half or be able to take on ten of the top ninja artists at once to be physically fit. Check out the activity level of those in the U.S.A. Only 26 percent of U.S. adults engage in vigorous leisure-time physical activity three or more times per week (defined as periods of vigorous physical activity lasting 10 minutes or more). About 59 percent of adults do no vigorous physical activity at all in their leisure time.[1] About 25 percent of young people (age 12 to 21) participate in light-to-moderate activity (e.g., walking, bicycling) nearly every day. About 50 percent regularly engage in vigorous physical activity. Approximately 25 percent report no vigorous physical activity, and 14 percent report no recent vigorous or light-to-moderate physical activity.[2] People drive just to go one block, for crying aloud. Are you kidding me? Do you really have to wonder why we are unhealthy? Does it surprise you that the percentage of overweight individuals is continuing to rise?

A Nielsen report released on September 29, 2005 stated that the average household in the United States watched eight hours and eleven minutes of television a day, the highest level since Nielsen first measured TV viewing in the '50s.[3] Do you find that as disturbing as I do? If I had to guess, many of these TV watchers are the same people who claim they have tried everything to lose weight and cannot. Understand that there are no quick or effortless solutions to people's weight problems—they have to commit to improving their life to change their health. If these

1. Lethbridge-Çejku M, Vickerie J. Summary health statistics for U.S. adults: National Health Interview Survey, 2003. National Center for Health Statistics. Vital Health Stat 10(225). 2005.

2. U.S. Department of Health and Human Services. Physical Activity and Health: A Report of the Surgeon General. Centers for Disease Control and Prevention. 1996.

3. "Nielsen Reports Americans Watch TV at Record Levels," NEW YORK, September 29, 2005—*Nielsen Media Research.*.

people turned off the TV and moved a little more, they would be singing a different song—the song of health. Do not kid yourself—take responsibility. Either you want to make changes or you do not. Did you watch the *Star Wars* movies? Yoda, the little green Jedi master, said, "there is no try, there is only *do* or do *not*." One of the easiest adjustments to make is to turn off the TV, because almost anything else uses more energy than watching the tube. You have the right to remain fat, or the choice to become fit. Which do you choose? *Get that monkey off your back!*

The television is not the only offender contributing to the United States' weight problem; modern conveniences such as the elevator, dishwasher, and even the TV remote control "save" upwards of 110 calories a day. Since introducing these conveniences, most people have not made lifestyle changes (decreased calorie consumption or increased movement) to compensate; hence, their weight has gone up. Take control of the situation—put down the remote, take the stairs, and wash your dishes!

Along with a well-balanced eating plan, exercise is important for losing and maintaining weight as well as preserving overall health. The National Weight Control Registry tells us that regular exercise is the key to *maintaining* weight, and for the first time ever the USDA's food pyramid includes exercise (MyPyramid.gov). In the nutrition chapter, I wrote that you must manage calories *in* versus calories *out*, and exercise definitely helps manage the calories "out."

When you exercise, you recharge your body by getting oxygen and blood flowing. As you become more physically fit, your heart will not have to work as hard during exercise or at rest. You will feel an overall improvement in your health and increase your longevity. In addition, prolonged, continuous exercise contributes to an increased production and release of endorphins, resulting in a sense of euphoria better known as "runner's high." Clearly, there is only an upside to exercise, so make it a habit!

Cardiovascular and weight-bearing exercises like weight training, walking or jogging help joints and muscles, help relieve or reduce arthritis pain, strengthen bones, and help decrease the risk for lifestyle-related diseases. Exercise can reduce stress, improve sleep, lower blood pressure, reduce the risk of fatal blood clots, decrease cardiovascular risk, and extend your lifespan. Exercise (and ultimately better health) can increase energy, body image, and sex drive. When you feel healthy and look better, chances are you will be more comfortable having sex. Many men and women complain about looking fat in front of their partners and are therefore embarrassed during sex or stop having sex all together; you have the power to change this if it has happened to you. Sex should be comfortable and enjoyable, so please do not allow your weight to hinder what should be a wonderful experience.

Benefits of exercise:

Increased metabolism: Calorie burning increases, aiding in weight loss or weight control. Exercised muscles burn calories and do so for several hours after the workout is completed.

Improved health: Your cardiovascular system (another name for the circulatory system, consisting of the heart, blood, and blood vessels) carries oxygen and nutrients to various parts of the body. Exercise improves how your heart, lungs, and muscles work together. Exercise gives you more energy and will improve your physical well-being. Aerobic exercise increases your cardiovascular fitness, endurance, and stamina. Your heart is a hard-working muscle and responds to exercise by becoming stronger and more efficient.

The lymphatic system is a specialized component of the circulatory system and is an important part of its defense against disease and combating foreign bodies such as viruses, bacteria, or fungi. The lymphatic system consists of: bone marrow, spleen, thymus gland, lymph nodes, tonsils, appendix, and a few other organs. Unlike your circulatory system that comes equipped with a pump (your heart), the lymphatic system does not. It is stimulated by muscle expansion and contraction; hence, it moves only as much as you. Therefore, the more you move, the more your body moves the lymph. Exercise results in a general improvement in bodily function, combined with improved lymphatic flow and increased immune hormonal balance.

Psychological well-being: The entire nervous system (for example, areas of the brain that control pleasure and elation) is stimulated during exercise. Numerous studies have shown that exercise increases alertness and IQ. While researchers have long touted exercise as a way to maintain physical fitness and help prevent high blood pressure, diabetes, obesity and other diseases, now a number of studies show that exercise also helps improve symptoms of certain mental conditions, including depression and anxiety.

Scientists believe that exercise may activate neurotransmitters (a chemical substance that transmits nerve impulses across a synapse) associated with pleasure and tension relief, such as serotonin, norepinephrine, and dopamine, creating a "brain cocktail" that puts us in a state in which we feel alert and calm. The term "runner's high" refers to this activation of neurotransmitters.

Regular exercise can be an extraordinary means of preventing or treating mild-to-moderate depression. Various studies have shown that the more someone exercises, the less likely he or she is to be depressed. It can therefore be an effective deterrent to stress, depression, and anxiety. If it does not eliminate the need for medication, perhaps it can help reduce the dosages that some individuals may currently be taking (consult with your physician).

Exercise also can be an excellent stress reducer. Stress manifests itself in the form of muscular tension and hormonal imbalances. Exercise releases the tension in muscles and stimulates the hormonal system.

Muscular stimulation: Exercising increases the circulation to the muscles, makes the muscles stronger, and makes the connective tissue stronger. Other benefits include improved physique, balance, and posture.

Skeletal stimulation: Research shows that bones become weaker if you do not stress them. Weight bearing cardiovascular exercises and strength training exercises has been shown to reduce osteoporosis. Exercise helps prevent bone calcium loss and helps maintain healthy bones.

Improved digestion: Exercise assists the natural peristaltic action (the waves of involuntary muscle contractions that transport food, waste matter, or other contents through a tube-shaped organ such as the intestine). Aaaahhhh, regularity!

Increased self-confidence: When you exercise and strengthen the body as a whole, you strengthen your mind as well. When you feel good physically, you will feel good about yourself. Watch and see what happens: You will hold your head higher and have a more confident stride.

Where to start

The American Council on Exercise advises getting into an exercise routine gradually but consistently. Please consult with your doctor if you are starting an exercise program for the first time. Incorporate simple lifestyle changes such as walking more and climbing stairs instead of taking the elevator (this will introduce movement spontaneously). Eventually you will aim for two hundred minutes a week, which is only forty minutes five days a week. You can break it up into two twenty-minute workouts in a day, or even four ten-minute workouts in a day. Regardless of how you decide to get moving, you will realize how undemanding it is. A twenty-minute weight training session at lunch and a twenty-minute walk after dinner is feasible, but work yourself up to this—do not get discouraged. Get out and move!

In order to achieve this goal, you must start moving. Everyone enjoys different activities, so figure out what works for you. Do you prefer to work out alone, or with other people? Do you like team sports? Do you like adventure? Are you more modest? Are you self-motivated, or do you need the structure of a class or a trainer? Some of you may find that you enjoy outdoor workouts and would be more inclined to hike or mountain bike. You can take that dance class you have always wanted to try.

You do not have to spend a fortune to exercise. You can buy simple, effective equipment for less than $100. For example: exercise bands of different resistances, tubing, medicine balls, rubber mats, jump ropes, and dumbbells are all inexpensive but effective. Please invest in the proper shoes to reduce the chance of injury.

You do not have to keep your cardio workouts isolated to machines. Take dance classes, go hiking, swimming, bicycling, or practice yoga—whatever keeps you moving and your heart rate elevated. Go power walking or Rollerblading, if that is what you enjoy. Play team sports like basketball, soccer, volleyball, or tennis. Get some workout videos and try something different. There is no "right" activity. You will find that trying something new—even something scary—can empower you and build self-confidence. I prefer to take dance classes or go running or walking at the beach. I also enjoy going to the gym and taking challenging classes from instructors who motivate me and seeing other people working hard. It does not matter how you do it—you just have to do it. You have to get off your couch and move, for the sake of your health. Stop making excuses, and start fitting movement into your day. Everyone gets busy—that is not a valid excuse; as I said before, exercise needs to be a priority. Exercising really can be a lot of fun, especially when it includes activities such as dancing, tennis, Frisbee, canoeing, skiing, squash, softball, base-ball, basketball, biking, or any other exciting activity. Even gardening and cleaning your house will burn calories. Stop wasting time watching TV, talking on the phone, and dillydallying, and instead get moving! Laziness will not get you the results you want! Tell yourself you will do it—and do it!

Many people ask me which activity burns the most calories. You do not need to work yourself into agonizing pain to increase cardiovascular strength, but you have to move. The activity that will burn the most calories will be the activity that you can spend the most time doing, or the activity in which you can push yourself the hardest. When it comes to equipment, the same applies. It does not matter which one burns more calories; what does matter is which machine *you* prefer. The bot-tom line is that the activity or machine you stay at the longest is the one that is going to burn the most calories (you want to enjoy yourself, so do not think about calories).

As far as cardiovascular equipment is concerned, I suggest that you try them all: the elliptical trainer, bicycle, Stairmaster, StepMill, rowing machine, treadmill, and Versa Climber are just some of the many choices you have. You may find that you like three or four different machines, thereby allowing for more variety in your workouts. You can even mix and match your workouts; for example, fifteen minutes on the elliptical, fifteen minutes on the bike, and fifteen minutes on the treadmill, and you can also mix up the speeds and incline levels to give yourself variation. Please, do not pay attention to the number of calories that the machine says you are burning, because the machine can be off by as much as 20–30 percent in either direction. Instead, focus on the intensity and time of your workouts.

Please—do not buy into the idea that you burn more calories or fat on an empty stomach. Weight loss is dependent upon overall calories burned, and you will have more energy to burn more calories if you have eaten something. There is a lot of time between your last meal of the day and when you wake up; therefore, it is essential to start the engine with some fuel. You have a choice in the morning: you can eat breakfast and kick your metabolism into gear, or you can skip breakfast and force your body to slow its metabolism down so you can work out. Breakfast is the most important meal of the day, which you should never sacrifice. You will naturally have more energy and stamina if you work out after you have eaten something.

In order to start your new program, you must be willing to put yourself first. *You* are the most important person—even if you have a wife, husband, partner, or child. This will require you to be selfish—and that is OK. You cannot put everyone else's needs before yours; you must take care of *you*. You have to learn to fit in "you time," because you are of no use to anyone else if you are weak, unhealthy, or tired. You will look better, and most importantly, you will feel better and when you feel your best, you will be able to give so much more of yourself. The happier you are, the happier everyone around you will be. It is OK to ask for the support of loved ones to assist you in starting and sticking to a regimen, because when you have a supportive cast the process of making lifestyle changes can be much easier.

To make fitness a permanent part of your lifestyle, choose activities that you love. Do not cross your fingers hoping for something to happen and stick. Turn off the TV, get off that couch, and make them happen. To stick with your exercise regimen, make sure that you are setting yourself up for success. Select *your* right time of day to work out because every person's "clock" is different. Most gyms offer inexpensive childcare services, so do not let that be an excuse. If you plan ahead and set expectations for yourself and others by announcing your schedule and by putting them into your day planner, computer, or calendar, it will allow you to stick to your program. Think of these scheduled workouts as you would any other important meeting that you should not miss. The loved ones in your life will understand your need to take time out of your day for your health. Keep a journal to track your progress (see Table 10).

Another method to help you stick to your program and keep you motivated is the use of the Internet. You can use the Internet to find workout partners, emotional support, and nutritional and exercise information. People place ads on sites like Craigslist in search of a workout partner(s). Other sites peertrainers.com, rockclimbing.com, sandeaters.org, sportsvite.com, yoplayas.com, and myactivitymatch.com; see if one of these sites can work for you. You will find it is embarrassing and very difficult to stand people up. Having a partner or a trainer holds you accountable, and you will most likely stick with your program.

Make your workout more efficient by avoiding distractions at the gym like magazines, the television, or the person next to you (unless they are helping you), and focus on your goal: your workout. Distractions cause you to work out less intensely, and that is self-defeating. You can use music as a motivator and let it help keep you focused. Studies show that fast-paced music increases workout intensity—definitely makes a difference for me. I will admit that I love to have a gossipy magazine to read to get me through my cardio workouts, but I stay focused on intensity and time. Make sure whatever you do, you do not compromise the intensity and purpose of your workout; otherwise, it may take you much longer to see results.

Make sure you also incorporate a weight-training program into your routine. Muscle is almost twice as dense as fat. Even though muscle weighs more than fat, fat makes you look bigger. Furthermore, muscle is metabolically active, so it requires more calories just to exist, whereas fat is metabolically lazy. Do you want to be a burning machine? The more muscle you have, the greater your calorie-burning potential, both at rest and when active! Strength training will become even more crucial as you hit your forties; because pumping iron will help you build and maintain muscle mass, help combat osteoporosis, increase energy, and improve balance.

When weight training, you must lift enough weight to challenge your muscles. I do suggest that you hire a personal trainer who can show you the proper techniques and help you get the results you want without compromising your safety. Once you feel you are comfortable with your routine, you can go off on your own. To start, you will usually be doing two to three sets of ten to fifteen repetitions. It is a myth to think that you can magically melt fat from one specific area, better known as spot reduction; the fat will naturally come off certain areas first—just be patient. As you become more experienced, you will be amazed at the variety of ways to work a muscle group; there are so many different exercises as well as techniques. I learn new ones almost every day, either by watching other personal trainers or reading about them in fitness magazines. There are plenty of publications with great descriptions and depictions of exercises, and I suggest you start reading some of them. I recommend *Men's Health, Men's Journal, Health, Fitness, Shape, Natural Health, Experience Life,* and *Yoga.*

There will be the people who go to the extreme and do too much exercise. This can be counterproductive and potentially dangerous. Most people cannot physically or mentally sustain going to the gym for two hours every day—they will burn out. Working out in this manner will set you up for overuse injuries, be side lined, and lose ground. Remember—your workouts are not a substitute for healthy eating. If you are constantly eating too much and going to the gym to burn off the calories, then you are setting yourself up for disappointment. Exercise, like eating, requires balance.

As with many things, we wish for immediate results. It will take time to see muscle tone and improvements in cardiovascular health. I promise you will see them. You will notice as time progresses that your stamina improves, your clothes fit better, you simply feel healthier, and you will be lowering most of your health risks, so keep on keeping on! Remember that the slower the weight comes off, the easier it is to maintain. This is usually because you are losing weight by healthy methods instead of crash diets that are impossible to maintain and sustain.

Some of you may be saying, "I'm too old to start working out." Do not deny yourself the chance to feel better. I have had clients in their late sixties start an exercise program, and they have seen tremendous results. My mother did not start working out in a gym until she was in her fifties. She loves to take yoga and Pilates and kick butt on the elliptical machine. Do you think that for a moment I was not going to do everything I could to encourage my mother to get into the best shape of her life? My father has also joined an incredible gym that allows him to increase his cardiovascular strength and stamina. He does a combination of different cardio machines and circuit training. You can be a hot mama or papa at any age. Tell yourself you are strong and capable, get yourself on an exercise program, and feel the change. You will love yourself for it! You will feel empowered.

It is important that you stay challenged if you want to stay motivated and continue to see results. Going through the motions is not enough. From time to time, it is a good idea to gain a fresh perspective and freshen up your routine by hiring a personal trainer. Your body is your machine for you to fine-tune. Be sure to get sufficient rest. Your body repairs itself at rest, so allow your body sufficient time to repair. Everyone's "sufficient time" will be different. I absolutely need 8 hours of sleep to function at my best. Love your body and keep it in its best condition! Respect your body.

As I mentioned in the nutrition chapter, it is important to change your calorie intake as you lose weight. For example, if you are a 200-pound female who does not exercise, you need approximately 2,460 calories simply to maintain your weight. If you are a 200-pound female who exercises lightly, you need 2,860 calories to maintain your weight. So, say you have been exercising lightly and now weigh 155 pounds; you would only need 2,217 calories to maintain your weight. This is why many people plateau, so be sure to make the necessary calorie adjustments. You can figure this out by visiting:

- www.bcm.edu/cnrc/caloriesneed.htm
- www.cancer.org/docroot/PED/content/PED_6_1x_Calorie_Calculator.asp
- www.primusweb.com/fitnesspartner/jumpsite/calculat.htm.
- For additional sites Google, *calorie calculator*.

Believing that you can do this is half the battle. Be positive and try your best, but you have to try. No one is going to do this for you—no magic pill or any other malarkey—only you, working consistently! Write down your training goals, and keep them in plain sight so that you have to read them every day (tape them to the mirror in your bathroom or your refrigerator). Exercising is not a free ticket to pigging out—everything in moderation! Additionally, remember to prioritize! It is important that you tackle one behavior at a time. Get moving, and get that monkey *off* your back!

Benefits of exercise: The heart is the most important muscle in the body, and exercise keeps it strong.

- Keeps resting heart rate low
- Oxygen is used more efficiently
- Energy levels increase
- Increased endurance
- Lower blood pressure
- Reduced risk of developing diabetes and other diseases
- Increase in good cholesterol, decrease in bad cholesterol
- More efficient cardiovascular system
- Reduced body fat and improved weight control
- Builds stronger bones and muscles
- Improved self-esteem and body image
- Better chance of maintaining a healthy weight throughout life
- Increased sex-drive
- Relieve stress
- Helps reduce depression and anxiety
- Helps improve psychological well-being

Table 9:
No Excuses! Stay Challenged! Don't Overdo It! Believe You Can
and Do! Excuse Busters.

Excuse	Buster
1. I am too tired	If you're physically tired, then go to bed and get a good night's rest. Then get up in the morning and get started. You have two choices: be tired after a day of successful exertion, or be tired after a day of zero movement. The choice is yours. If you're going to be tired anyway, wouldn't it make sense to get something out of it? Burn some calories. Take action in the direction of your goal, you'll find that it can be invigorating.
2. I do not have time	If this is your excuse, I will assume you do not watch any television, surf the Web, or talk on the phone. You have to want to make exercise a priority in your life. You do not have to kill yourself to reap the benefits of exercise. Replace an hour of TV viewing with an hour workout—go for a walk, run, bike ride, etc. Find something that will fit into your schedule and enjoy the benefits. You do not have to go to a gym to reap the benefits of a good workout. Do anything more than you were doing before.

3. It is boring	It doesn't have to be. Spice things up and find activities you love that will stick. Change your activity frequently to avoid burnout.
4. Comparing yourself with others	This is unrealistic and will lead to feelings of insignificance. Instead, set challenging, but attainable, goals and focus on how *you* feel each time you achieve them. Celebrate your successes with a manicure, new shoes, tickets to a ball game, a golf club, a new CD or *iTunes* download.

➢ **Focus on strength, flexibility, cardiovascular endurance, and your overall health!** Mood is ultimately the key to staying on course. Start thinking positively and commit to be fit! Make exercise a daily priority.

Here are some calorie burning ideas:
- Turn off the TV!
- Strap on a pedometer and keep track of how much you are walking in a day
- Walk up stairs rather than using elevators or escalators
- Scrub the pots by hand
- Pace while on the phone
- Park far from the entrance when you shop
- Use public transport and walk to the station or bus stop

- Go for a walk
- Mow the lawn
- Rake leaves
- Play with the kids
- Join a walking group in the neighborhood or at the local shopping mall
- Recruit a partner for support and encouragement
- Take a walk after dinner (if it's cold, bundle up)
- Do some gardening—pull weeds
- Put some music on and shake what your mama gave you
- Cook your meals (standing and stirring burns calories)
- Clean the house—vacuum, clean the floors and baseboards, etc.
- Walk the dog (if you have one, or get one)
- Wash and wax your car by hand
- Help shovel the snow when it snows
- Paint the walls
- Go window-shopping
- Do errands by bike or foot
- Jump rope
- Get a hobby that makes you move
- Get up from your desk and take a walk
- Clean out your closet
- Chop some wood for a fire
- Gather all your old stuff to sell on eBay
- Replace a coffee break with a brisk ten-minute walk
- Have sex

Let Me Repeat: Why Exercise Is So Great

1. Increased metabolism
2. Decreased resting heart rate
3. Altered cholesterol levels
4. Neural stimulation
5. Muscular stimulation
6. Skeletal stimulation
7. Improved digestion
8. Improved lymphatic flow
9. Reduced stress
10. Increased immune-system/ resistance (better resistance to disease)
11. Weight control
12. Increased fat burning
13. Improved endurance
14. Increased strength
14. Increased muscle mass
15. Increased joint mobility
16. Improved cardiovascular fitness
17. Improved energy levels and increased general stamina
18. Better sleep
19. Psychological benefits—exercise improves mood, reduces depression and anxiety
20. Better Sex

Table 10:
Exercise Log.

1. **Exercise:** What type of movement did you incorporate today?

2. **Length of time:** How long did you exercise?

3. **What was your intensity level:** On a scale of 1-10 (ten being the most vigorous) what was your energy output?

4. **How did you feel during your workout?** Were you having fun or did you want it to be over with before you even started? Did you pick an exercise that was fun? How did your body feel? Any aches and pains? Were these serious pains or just soreness from a new activity?

5. **How did you feel after your workout?** Some people try to do too much too soon and get sore and frustrated and do not want to continue. Pay attention to how you feel, so you can stay motivated. You will feel some level of soreness, especially if you are just starting a program, but you should not push yourself to the point that you cannot walk for a week after.

6. **Review each week:** How much movement did you incorporate this week? What can you do in order to add more movement?

Chapter Ten

Are You Ready, Willing, and Able?

"I understand and realize the emphasis on being motivated by how we look, but I have gotten so connected to the idea of how we *feel* about how we look…. Life can't be all about looks. We have to be searching for something greater in order to even enjoy how we look."
~Gabrielle Reece

"You choose … whether to give up at first obstacle or give it your all, to speak up or stay silent, to change what you don't like or let it change you. With every word, every step you take, you define who you are— and create your future."
~Fitness Magazine, November 2005

"No matter how many times you fail at something, you are never a failure until the day you quit trying."
~Michael T. Vaisanen

There is a serious problem concerning personal health in this country. *The Land of the Plenty* is certainly living up to its reputation regarding food consumption. We are jeopardizing our health, and to make this problem worse, there is a new diet book published and on the bookstore shelves nearly every month. These "diet" books fail to address the real underlying issues and fail to help their readers make lasting lifestyle changes.

Stop the dieting nonsense! *Eat that monkey!* A one-size-fits-all diet will not lead to a healthier life or permanent weight loss. You can achieve these things only by first understanding yourself and by understanding your patterns concerning food and exercise. Only then will you understand what healthful eating and exercise are really about for *you*!

Gain control of your life and your weight. Most importantly—get healthy! It is time to take the power back by acknowledging your monkey and challenging him head on with a real understanding of yourself, nutrition, and exercise. I want you to learn how easy it really is to add movement into your life. I want you to feel good about making the right food choices, all the time and for the right reasons. I want you to make small adjustments and allow them to become habits before tackling another. I want you to be healthy and reap the resulting lifestyle rewards. I want you to *eat your monkey*!

The diet books that have been or are currently on the market cover related subjects; however, they all go back to the "diet"—this is what you must eat for the next two weeks so that you can lose twenty pounds. It may be that creating a "diet" sells more books; however, this strategy is not realistic, and its results are temporary.

I want the "dieting" to stop. I want people to understand their behaviors and ask themselves why they are unhealthy. I want people to understand that permanent weight loss is possible, but they have to make permanent behavioral and psychological changes.

Eat that Monkey does not speak in "diet" terms. *Eat that Monkey* seeks to address the root cause of the problem, not the symptom.

You have made the first step to changing your life by picking up this book and reading it; now you have to apply the principles. Are you ready? Are you truly ready to make changes in your eating habits and exercise habits? Are you willing? Are you willing to give up fried foods for grilled foods, full sugar sodas for diet soda or water, candy for fruit? Are you able? Come on and face it—everyone is able. Do you have the desire to change? It is your choice. Making lifestyle changes will take time and effort. You must make the commitment and set realistic goals.

You must enjoy this process. Do not look at eating well and exercising as just a way to lose weight. When you eat better and exercise, you will feel more connected to your body. This amazing journey will change your life forever. You will find your true beauty and the athlete inside.

Make the choice to change old patterns of eating, non-exercise, and negative thinking. You have the power not to feel guilty, discouraged, or cynical. Rid yourself of your monkey and become liberated. Start practicing positive thinking!

Set a realistic long-term goal (your vision); then achieve it by reaching smaller, short-term goals by prioritizing the behaviors that are most in need of change. Focus on each day; eventually you will reach your ultimate goal. Remember, all foods, if eaten in moderation, can be a part of a healthy diet. The principal authority on your weight is what and how much you eat, not when you eat. Weight is contingent on the balance of calories consumed versus calories burned. Take in more calories than your body needs, and you gain weight. Take in less, and you lose weight. The time of day you consume these calories is not relevant.

Work yourself into your workouts. Take one day at a time, and stay true to yourself and your goal(s). Remember the basis of your success will be on improving personal performance—for yourself. Keep your focus by addressing the immediate benefits of making lifestyle changes, and looking better in the future will be a natural result. Change is a process that you must commit to every day.

A conscious assessment of your goals, your behavior, your relationships, and your performance in all areas ultimately enables self-improvement. It allows you to expand your options in life. Be honest when assessing your self! It can be painful. Confront yourself; only then can you seriously work to change what you can. You have the power to change how you spend your time, how you eat and drink, and personal performance. Analyze your performance while accepting yourself. Aim to change poisonous behavior today. Visualization is powerful. Visualize how you want to look and feel. Create an image of your optimal self and reach that goal. I cannot emphasize enough that you should prioritize your changes—do not attempt to change multiple behaviors at the same time—work on one behavior at a time.

Just Say YES!

- I truly have the *Desire* to lead a healthful life
- *I Choose*
- I will write down my *Goals*
- I will make the *Changes* necessary to achieve success
- I will take *Responsibility for my Actions*
- I will be in *Control*
- I will use *Positive Word*
- I will *Succeed*

Each of us has the Power of Choice, Change, Control, and Word. Use your power to change your life forever.

You *can* do this! Eat your monkey.

Visit www.eatthatmonkey.com for more support.

"Don't ever give up on a dream due to the amount of time it will take to achieve it. The time will pass anyway."
~Russ Ebsen

"True victory is not about finishing first; it is about finishing regardless of how many times you fall."
~Rebecca Eilts

"To begin a journey one must have courage; to finish a journey one must have perseverance."
~Alex Sung

"There never was a winner that didn't expect to win in advance."
~Denis Waitley

"The greatest success is not giving up, even when it seems like you should. When things seem unclear, I sit back and ask myself, where are you going and what do you need to do right now to get there?"
~Joseph Magagnoli

Eat that Monkey seminars

Erica Porter has been a health and fitness enthusiast and participant her entire life—from gymnast, swimmer, dancer, and professional wrestler to educating others as a personal trainer, health and fitness consultant, lifestyle and weight management specialist, and lifestyle motivator. These combined experiences have given Erica a keen understanding of the human body and psyche, creating a profound aspiration to enlighten and inspire achievement of optimal health and superior well-being.

Erica has had the opportunity to educate many people over the years. As she analyzed the symptom of poor health looking for ways to affect lasting change for her clients, it became obvious that unhappiness in any form could manifest itself in dangerous and destructive lifestyle habits. After witnessing many of her clients and acquaintances make lasting and positive health changes under her guidance, Erica realized that she must leverage her ability so as to benefit as many people as possible. Answering for everyone, what individuals have been asking her for years … how do I achieve lasting good health? This is what compelled Erica to write *Eat That Monkey, Now Is the Time to Change Your Life!* and to create her powerful Choose, Change, Control seminars. Erica's focus is on encouraging the masses to take responsibility for their "self" and their life. Erica motivates and facilitates positive lifestyle changes and creates the perspective required for healthy daily living.

Erica is versatile, professional, knowledgeable, funny and charismatic, and her expertise and life experience can guide you to accomplishing your most important and elusive goals. Erica shares her secrets for expanding personal growth and becoming genuinely satisfied with your life. Her success as an educator, athlete, and professional speaker, coupled with her genuine optimism and enthusiasm make every presentation a starting point for personal and professional growth. Her messages are always personal, interactive, and entertaining for large and small audiences alike. Erica Porter is the consummate presenter whose distinguished physical appearance commands credibility.

Based on your group's needs and preferences, Erica will create a customized presentation, incorporating material from one or more of her signature topics—Lifestyle, Performance, Change, Leadership.

Erica D. Porter
www.EatThatMonkey.com

Notes

Chapter One

1. National Diabetes Information Clearinghouse, http://diabetes.niddk. nih.gov/dm/pubs/statistics/index.htm#14 Cost of Diabetes in the United States, 2002

- Total (direct and indirect): $132 billion.
- Direct medical costs: $92 billion.
- Indirect costs (related to disability, work loss, premature death): $40 billion.
- Average annual health care costs for a person *with* diabetes: $13,243.
- Average annual health care costs for a person *without* diabetes: $2,560.

2. American Heart Association, www.americanheart.org

Everybody has—and needs—blood pressure. Without it, blood can't circulate through the body. And without circulating blood, vital organs can't get the oxygen and food that they need to work. So it's important to know about blood pressure and how to keep it within a healthy level. Normal blood pressure falls within a range; it's not one set of numbers.

When the heart beats, it pumps blood to the arteries and creates pressure in them. This pressure (<u>blood pressure</u>) results from two forces. The first force is created as blood pumps into the arteries and through the circulatory system. The second is created as the arteries resist the blood flow.

If you're healthy, your arteries are muscular and elastic. They stretch when your heart pumps blood through them. How much they stretch depends on how much force the blood exerts.

Your heart beats about 60 to 80 times a minute under normal conditions. Your blood pressure rises with each heartbeat and falls when your heart relaxes between beats. Your blood pressure can change from minute to minute, with changes in posture, exercise or sleeping, **but it should normally be less than 120/80 mm Hg for an adult.** Blood pressure that stays between 120–139/80–89 is considered prehypertension and above this level (140/90 mm Hg or higher) is considered high (hypertension). Your doctor may take several readings over time before deciding whether your blood pressure is high.

What do blood pressure numbers indicate?

- The higher (systolic) number represents the pressure while the heart is beating.

- The lower (diastolic) number represents the pressure when the heart is resting between beats.

The systolic pressure is always stated first and the diastolic pressure second. For example: 118/76 (118 over 76); systolic = 118, diastolic = 76.

High blood pressure is a lifelong disease. It can usually be controlled but not cured. Once you begin to manage it and start a treatment program, maintaining a lower blood pressure is easier. By controlling your high blood pressure, you'll lower your risk of diseases like stroke, heart attack, heart failure, and kidney disease. You **can** do it!

The first thing to do is to have your blood pressure checked. If you have high blood pressure, you can do a lot to reduce it. Work with your doctor to determine the best treatment for you.

- It may include reducing the fat (particularly saturated fat) in your diet, eating less salt, and changing your lifestyle by losing weight and getting regular physical activity.

- Quitting smoking is also important to reduce your overall risk for heart attack and stroke.

- Your doctor may recommend reducing how much alcohol you drink.

- Many medicines also can help reduce and control high blood pressure. Your doctor will decide whether you need medicine in addition to dietary and lifestyle changes.

3. American Heart Association, www.americanheart.org

The American Heart Association has identified several risk factors. Some of them can be modified, treated or controlled, and some can't. The more risk factors you have, the greater your chance of developing coronary heart disease. Also, the greater the level of each risk factor, the greater the risk. For example, a person with a total cholesterol of 300 mg/dL has a greater risk than someone with a total cholesterol of 245 mg/dL, even though everyone with a total cholesterol greater than 240 is considered high-risk.

What are the major risk factors that can't be changed?
Increasing age
Male sex (gender)
Heredity (including race)

What are the major risk factors you can modify, treat or control by changing your lifestyle or taking medicine?
Tobacco smoke
High blood cholesterol
High blood pressure
Physical inactivity
Obesity and overweight
Diabetes Mellitus

What other factors contribute to heart disease risk?
Stress
Alcohol

4. Wolf, A.M., and Colditz, G.A. Current estimates of the economic cost of obesity in the United States. Obesity Research 6(2):97-106, 1998.

Chapter Three

1. EDReferral.com (eating disorder referral.com), "Famous celebrities who have spoken publicly about their suffering with Eating Disorders," December 1, 2006.

2. Princess of Wales, Interview by Martin Bashir, BBC News, available online http://www.bbc.co.uk/politics97/diana/panorama.html, September 14, 2006.

3. "Celebrities and the media, the pressure to be thin," http://www.eating-disorder-information.com/mediacelebrities.asp, November 20, 2006, accessed on February 19, 2007.

Chapter Four

1. Katherine M. Flegal, PhD; Barry I. Graubard, PhD; David F. Williamson, PhD; Mitchell H. Gail, MD, PhD, "Excess Deaths Associated With Underweight, Overweight, and Obesity," Vol. 293 No. 15, April 20, 2005, *Journal of the American Medical Association.*

2. Ogden CL, Carroll MD, Curtin LR, McDowell MA, Tabak CJ, Flegal KM. Prevalence of overweight and obesity in the United States, 1999–2004. *Journal of the American Medical Association.* 2006; 295:1549–1555.

3. *Preventing Obesity and Chronic Diseases Through Good Nutrition and Physical Activity,* http://www.cdc.gov/nccdphp/publications/factsheets/Prevention/obesity.htm, February 21, 2006.

4. R. Sturm, "The Effects of Obesity, Smoking, and Drinking on Medical Problems and Costs," *Health Affairs* (Mar/Apr 2002): 245–253.

5. Eric Schlosser, *Fast Food Nation: The Dark Side of the American Meal*, Boston: Houghton Mifflin, 2001. pg. 240.

6. Jonathan Rowe, "The Growth Consensus Unravels," paragraph 18, *Dollars & Sense The Magazine of Economic Justice*.

7. Gary Gardner and Brian Halweil, *Overfed and Underfed: The Global Epidemic of Malnutrition, Worldwatch Institute, pg. 32,* Michael F. Jacobson, "Liquid Candy: How Soft Drinks are Harming Americans' Health" (Washington, DC: CSPI, October 1998); Brian Wansink, "Can Package Size Accelerate Usage Volume?" *Journal of Marketing*, July 1996; Lisa R. Young and Marion Nestle, "Variation in Perceptions of a 'Medium' Food Portion: Implications for Dietary Guidance," *Journal of the American Dietetic Association*, April 1998.
    Among the newest marketing strategies is the "supersizing" of french fries, popcorn, pizzas, soda, and other fast-food items—at little extra cost to the consumer. The standard 6.5-ounce soda container of the 1950s, for example, has been supplanted by 20-ounce bottles, and one U.S. convenience store pushes a 64-ounce, 600-calorie "Double Gulp" soda bucket. The extra food content costs manufacturers little, since the ingredients account for a tiny share of the sale price; the consumer is paying mostly for the brand name, packaging, and marketing. To the consumer, such a "good value" is highly enticing. But supersizing may be skewing peoples' conception of what a "normal" serving is: in 1998, surveyed Americans consistently labeled as "medium" portions that were double or triple the size of USDA's "medium" guidelines. And consumer behavior studies show that people consistently consume more when they eat from larger containers.

8. http://www.bk.com/#menu=3,-1,-1, February 26, 2007.

9. http://www.mcdonalds.com/app_controller.nutrition.index1.html, February 26, 2007.

10. Jane Hurley and Bonnie Liebman, "X-Treme Eating, increasingly indulgent menus entice diners to pig out," *Nutrition Action Healthletter*, March 2007, pg. 13.

11. Diane Martindale, *Burgers on the brain*, Article from New Scientist vol 177 issue 2380. Date: 1 February 2003.

12. Daily News Central, *FDA's Call for Smaller Restaurant Portions Draws Criticism*, 03 June, 2006 15:58 GMT, http://health.dailynewscentral.com/content/view/2279/63, February 20, 2007.

13. Advertising in United States from Anthony E. Gallo, "Food Advertising in the United States," in Elizabeth Frazao, ed., *America's Eating habits: Changes and Consequences* (Washington, DC: United States Department of Agriculture (USDA), Economic Research Service (ERS), April 1999.

14. Yafu Zhao, M.S. and William Encinosa, Ph.D, Bariatric Surgery Utilization and Outcomes in 1998 and 2004, Healthcare cost and utilization project, January 2007, pg. 1.

15. Sandra G. Boodman, "Who are you calling fat?" The Washington Post, July 18, 2006, F1 and F4.

16. Nanci Hellmich, "Third of kids tip the scales the wrong way," USA Today, April 15, 2006.

17. Sharon Mickle, "Snacks, Sodas—and Calories—Climbing in Kids," Food Surveys Research Group, http://www.ars.usda.gov/is/np/fnrb/fnrb1000.htm, February 21, 2007.
U.S. kids today are eating more food and more calories than kids did 20 years ago, according to the latest U.S. Department of Agriculture data on the food intakes of nearly 10,000 children nationwide. ARS nutritionists combined data from a special 1998 nationwide survey of 5,559

children from birth to 9 years old with those from the 1994-96 national survey (CSFII) of all age groups. The earlier survey included 4,253 children to age 9. Trends gleaned from the combined data generally concur with the 1994-96 findings.

Snacks contributed a significant percent of daily calories—around 20 percent, on average. Among the most frequently reported snacks for the ages 9 and under were milk, fruits, cookies, candies, crackers, popcorn, pretzels and corn chips. Eighty-three percent of kids snacked on the day surveyed—up from 65 percent in the 1977-78 survey.

Over the last two decades, soft drink consumption increased 21 percent among 2- to 5-year-olds and 37 percent among 6- to 9-year-olds. Both age groups also drank more fruit juices and fruit drinks—26 percent and 11 percent more, respectively. Milk consumption, on the other hand, dropped 4 percent among the preschoolers and 10 percent among the older group. Twice as many kids ate crackers, popcorn, pretzels and corn chips in the 90s as did kids in the 70s.

Chapter Five

1. Medline Plus Medical Encyclopedia, http://www.nlm.nih.gov/medlineplus/ency/article/001605.htm, February 21, 2007.

Prader-Willi syndrome is a congenital (present from birth) disease characterized by obesity, decreased muscle tone, decreased mental capacity, and hypogonadism. The growing child exhibits slow mental and delayed motor development, increasing obesity, and characteristically small hands and feet. Rapid weight gain may occur during the first few years because the patient develops uncontrollable hunger that leads to morbid obesity. Mental development is slow, and the IQ seldom exceeds 80. However, children with Prader-Willi generally are very happy, smile frequently, and are pleasant to be around. Affected children have an intense craving for food and will do almost anything to get it. This results in uncontrollable weight gain. Morbid obesity (the degree of obesity that seriously affects health) may lead to respiratory failure with hypoxia (low blood oxygen levels), cor pulmonale (right-sided heart failure), and death.

2. Medline Plus Medical Encyclopedia, http://www.nlm.nih.gov/
medlineplus/ency/article/000353.htm, February 21, 2007.

Hypothyroidism is a condition in which the thyroid gland fails to produce enough thyroid hormone. The thyroid gland, located in the front of the neck just below the larynx, secretes hormones that control metabolism. These hormones are thyroxine (T4) and triiodothyronine (T3). The secretion of T3 and T4 is controlled by the pituitary gland and the hypothalamus, which is part of the brain. Thyroid disorders may result not only from defects in the thyroid gland itself, but also from abnormalities of the pituitary or hypothalamus. Hypothyroidism, or underactivity of the thyroid gland, may cause a variety of symptoms and may affect all body functions. The body's normal rate of functioning slows, causing mental and physical sluggishness and weight gain. The symptoms may vary from mild to severe.

Chapter Seven

1. Matthew Herper and Peter Kang, "The World's 10 Best Selling Drugs,"
Forbes.com, March 28, 2006.

2. Ritt Goldstein, "Drug Industry Scandal a 'Crisis,'" *Inter Press Service News Agency*, Oct. 4, 2004. Ashley Pringle (under Supervision from Dr. Chris McDonald, "Pharmaceutical Scandal or not? The Distinction Elaborated," www.pharmacoethics.com/categorization.html, February 21, 2007. Mike Adams, "Merck now under criminal investigation by the Justice Department for Vioxx scandal," *NewsTarget.com*, January 1, 2005.

3. American Heart Association, "Statistics you need to know-Statistics on Medication," http://www.americanheart.org/presenter.jhtml?identifier =107, February 21, 2007 (Source for medication statistics: The National Council on Patient Information and Education).

4. Jonathan Cohn, "Medicare Reform: The Real Winners, TNR: Insurance Companies, Drug Manufacturers Come Out Ahead," *The New Republic Story*, Nov. 20, 2003.

In fact, there's a long list of people—from insurance companies to prescription drug manufacturers—who got *exactly* what they wanted, and then some. Magically enough, they also happen to be groups that have spent a ton of money financing political campaigns and then lobbying the members they helped elect.

First on this list is the pharmaceutical industry. The Medicare compromise pumps $400 billion over ten years into the purchase of prescription drugs. Some of that money will simply displace money people already spend on their own, but much of it will be new money that would not otherwise have been spent. For the drug industry, that means more revenues and profits. But even more important here is what the government isn't doing: forcing down drug prices. Because private insurance companies, and not the government, will in theory be administering the benefit, the government won't have the power to bargain with drug makers the way that foreign governments do. Meanwhile, drug company lobbyists managed to gut a provision that would have legalized limited re-importation of drugs from Canada, where prescriptions cost less. Also gone is a proposal that would have eliminated some of the legal tricks drug makers use to thwart competition by generic manufacturers.

So the drug industry ends up with bigger sales but no pressure to lower its prices. Pretty sweet. Apparently that $22 million the industry spent on political contributions in 2002

5. Stephanie Saul, "Drug makers pay for lunch as they pitch," *The New York Times*, July 28, 2006, C1 and C7.

6. Maryann Napoli, "Many Prescription Drugs Have Unexpected Harmful Effects," *Center for Medical Consumers, Inc.*, May 2002. Gary Null PhD, Carolyn Dean MD ND, Martin Feldman MD, Debora Rasio MD, Dorothy Smith PhD, "Death by Medicine," 2003, entire document.

Chapter Eight

1. Frazao, E. "The high costs of poor eating patterns in the United States," in: Frazao, E., ed. *America's Eating Habits: Changes and*

Consequences. Washington, DC: U.S. Department of Agriculture (USDA), Economic Research Service (ERS), AIB-750, 1999.

Over the past several decades, dramatic changes in food purchasing and food preparation trends have occurred in the United States, including an increase in the number of meals eaten away from home and a decrease in time spent in meal preparation at home. Overall, households spent 38 percent of their food dollar on food eaten away from home in 1992. By comparison, in the 1970s, 20 percent of the food dollar was spent on food eaten away from home. This trend in meals eaten away from home shows no sign of weakening. In 1993, Americans spent $197.8 billion on meals eaten away from home, an increase of 9 percent above that in 1992. Currently, the restaurant industry as a whole is growing at a modest rate of 3 percent annually, whereas fast food restaurants are growing at a rate of 7 percent annually. The proliferation of fast food restaurants is evident in most parts of the country, there being an average of 1.02 fast food hamburger establishments/10,000 residents in the United States. The implications of more meals being eaten away from home on the nutritional quality of the diet are likely unfavorable. Although healthful food choices can be found at fast food restaurants, most foods available tend to contain undesirable amounts of energy and fat. A survey conducted by *Restaurants & Institutions* in 1994 found that consumers expressed increased interested in more healthful menu options, such as salads, grilled chicken, and fish; salads were found to be the second-most ordered food in restaurants. Of interest, hamburgers were found to be the most frequently ordered item, and French fries were the third-most ordered item.

Aside from eating more meals away from home, Americans appear to be spending less time preparing meals that are consumed at home. In 1987, 43 percent of all meals included at least one item made from scratch; in 1997, this value dropped to 38 percent. To meet consumer demands for foods that require minimal preparation time, supermarkets are increasing their selection of prepared foods. Along with offering convenience foods such as frozen dinners, supermarkets are offering precooked meals, such as rotisserie chicken, to better compete with restaurants.

Availability and sales of reduced-energy and reduced-fat products: In response to consumer interest in reducing dietary fat and energy intakes, a plethora of reduced-energy and reduced-fat food products has been introduced to the marketplace. Consumer acceptance of these products appears to be high. An estimated three-fourths of adults regularly consume reduced-fat foods. A study conducted to evaluate the size and growth of the market for nutritionally improved products between 1989 and 1993 used supermarket scanner data to track the growth in sales of these products relative to that of their traditional counterparts. Sales of nutritionally improved products, including reduced-energy and reduced-fat products, grew faster than did sales of traditional counterparts of these foods in the supermarkets included in this study.

Health concerns and a desire to reduce fat and energy intakes are the primary reasons consumers give for choosing reduced-energy and reduced-fat products. However, whether intakes of these foods actually lead to reduced fat and energy intakes has been questioned. Anecdotal observations suggest that consumers may not use reduced-energy and reduced-fat products as one-to-one substitutes for their traditional counterparts. It is possible that reduced-energy and reduced-fat products are being consumed in addition to rather than in place of other foods, thereby resulting in an increase rather than a decrease in energy and fat intakes. In addition, larger portions of reduced-energy and reduced-fat products are perhaps being consumed, thereby nullifying any beneficial effect of these products. Results of ongoing population-based studies evaluating the effects of reduced-energy and reduced-fat products on body weight and energy and fat intakes are not yet available. Thus, it is difficult to infer what the influence of increased availability of these products on trends in energy and fat intakes might be.

Changes in food-portion sizes: Anecdotal evidence suggests that food-portion sizes have been on the rise in recent years and may be increasing energy intakes. Scant data are available, however, regarding actual trends in portion sizes and potential implications of larger portions on food and nutrient intakes. The *National Restaurant Association* conducted a study in which menus collected in 1988 from sixty-six restaurants were compared with menus collected in 1993 from the same restaurants. The number of menus offering entrées with more than one portion size, such as "queen-size" and "king-size" steak, increased by 12 percent during this period.

2. Sherry Holetzky, "*What is metabolism,*" http://www.wisegeek.com/what-is-metabolism.htm, February 22, 2007.

The term *metabolism*, derived from the Greek language, simply means change or transformation. It relates to various processes within the body that convert food and other substances into energy and other metabolic byproducts used by the body. It is a necessary function that allows our bodies to use food and other resources to maintain the working parts, repair damage, heal injury and rid the body of toxins. In other words, metabolism is a necessary process, without which living organisms would die.

Metabolism aids in digestive function as well as absorption of nutrients. It is most affected by nutrition, hydration and physical activity. Each of these items is an imperative aspect of optimum metabolic health. When any one of these is lacking, the metabolic rate decreases. Consequently, weight loss and weight maintenance are directly related to healthy metabolism.

While lowering your calorie and fat intake may be important parts of weight loss, both decrease your metabolism. It is therefore essential to stimulate the metabolic rate through other means such as routine physical activity. It is not a good idea to skip meals or to reduce calories by an extreme amount, since decreased metabolism causes the body to burn fewer calories and less fat. It may also cause your body to store excess fat in reserve.

Metabolism is also the process the body uses to break down chemicals such as drugs. When you take medication, your body employs *catabolic* metabolism, to break down larger molecules into smaller ones that can be more readily absorbed. *Anabolic* metabolism is the opposite of catabolic. It uses enzymes to structure larger molecules from smaller ones.

The body utilizes the many complex processes that make up metabolism to facilitate physical function, assist growth, aid in healing and in essence, support life.

3. Dr. Paula Baillie-Hamilton, *Toxic Overload: A Doctor's Plan for Combating the Illnesses Caused by Chemicals in Our Foods, Our Homes, and Our Medicine Cabinets*, Part II The Chemical Connection to Chronic Illness, May 2005.

4. http://ask.yahoo.com/20020926.html, Definition: Free Radical, *Britannica Concise*, February 6, 2007.

Typically, stable molecules contain pairs of electrons. When a chemical reaction breaks the bonds that hold paired electrons together, free radicals are produced. Free radicals contain an odd number of electrons, which makes them unstable, short-lived, and highly reactive. As they combine with other atoms that contain unpaired electrons, new radicals are created, and a chain reaction begins. This process is essential for the decomposition of many different substances at high temperatures.

However, in the human body, oxidized free radicals are believed to cause tissue damage at the cellular level—harming our DNA, mitochondria, and cell membrane. An article titled "Antioxidants and Free Radicals" from the SportsMedWeb explains that *antioxidants* are molecules that defend the body from cellular damage by ending the free radical chain reaction before vital molecules are harmed. Sometimes referred to as "free radical scavengers," the most commonly recognized antioxidants are vitamin E, beta-carotene (a pre-cursor to vitamin A), and vitamin C. The trace metal selenium is required for the function of one of our antioxidant enzyme systems, and is often included in lists of antioxidant micronutrients (i.e., vitamins).

According to information we found on the web site of the Atlanta-based Edelson Center for Environmental and Preventive Medicine, the theory of <u>free radical pathology</u> was first proposed in the 1950s by Dr. Denham Harman, a professor emeritus at the University of Nebraska. Now considered the father of the <u>free-radical theory of aging</u>, Harman believes that we should reduce our intake of calories to decrease the incidence of disease.

Chapter Nine

1. Lethbridge-Çejku M, Vickerie J. 'Summary health statistics for U.S. adults: National Health Interview Survey," 2003. National Center for Health Statistics. Vital Health Stat 10(225). 2005.

2. U.S. Department of Health and Human Services. "Physical Activity and Health: A Report of the Surgeon General," Centers for Disease Control and Prevention, 1996.

3. "Nielsen Reports Americans Watch TV at Record Levels," New York, September 29, 2005—*Nielsen Media Research.*
    Nielsen Media Research reported today that the average American home watched more television the past TV season versus any previous season. During the 2004–05 TV season (which started September 20, 2004 and ended September 18, 2005), the average household in the United States tuned into television an average of eight hours and eleven minutes per day. This is 2.7 percent higher than the previous season, 12.5 percent higher than ten years ago, and the highest levels ever reported since television viewing was first measured by *Nielsen Media Research* in the 1950s. During the September 2004–September 2005 season, the average person watched television four hours and thirty-two minutes each day, the highest level in fifteen years (See Table 1). Household tuning levels going back to the 1950s can be downloaded at the following link: [http://www.nielsenmedia.com/newsreleases/2005/TVviewinglevels.xls].
    The day Primetime during the 2004–05 season saw a slight increase in viewing from the previous season (see Table 2).

Table 1

Average Hours: Minutes Tuned into TV Per 24 Hour Period

Broadcast Year (Sept-Sept)	Homes Avg. Hours: Minutes per day	Persons 2+ Avg. Hours: Minutes per day
2004–2005	8:11	4:32
2003–2004	8:01	4:25
2002–2003	7.55	4.25
2001–2002	7.42	4.18
2000–2001	7.39	4.15
1999–2000	7.31	4.06
1998–1999	7.24	4.00
1997–1998	7.15	3.58
1996–1997	7.12	3.56
1995–1996	7.15	3.59
1994–1995	7.15	4.02
1993–1994	7.16	4.03
1992–1993	7.12	4.06
1991–1992	7.05	4.06

Table 2

Average Hours: Minutes Tuned into TV During Primetime Each Day

Broadcast Year (Sept-Sept)	Homes Avg. Hours: Minutes Primetime	Persons 2+ Avg. Hours: Minutes Primetime
2004–2005	1:53	1:11
2003–2004	1:52	1:10
2002–2003	1:52	1:10
2001–2002	1:51	1:10
2000–2001	1:52	1:10
1999–2000	1:51	1:09
1998–1999	1:50	1:08
1997–1998	1:49	1:08
1996–1997	1:49	1:08
1995–1996	1:50	1:09
1994–1995	1:50	1:10
1993–1994	1:51	1:11
1992–1993	1:50	1:11
1991–1992	1:50	1:12

About Nielsen Media Research

Nielsen Media Research is the world's leading provider of television audience measurement and advertising information services. In the United States, Nielsen's *National People Meter* service provides audience estimates for all national program sources, including broadcast networks, cable networks, Spanish language networks, and national syndicators. Local ratings estimates are produced for television stations, regional cable networks, MSOs, cable interconnects, and Spanish language stations in each of the two hundred and ten television markets in the United States, including electronic metered service in fifty-six markets. For more information, please visit: www.nielsenmedia.com. *Nielsen Media Research* is part of *VNU Media Measurement & Information*, a global leader in information services for the media and entertainment industries. The group serves the information and marketing needs of television and radio broadcasters, advertisers, agencies, media planners, music companies, publishers, motion-picture studios, distributors and exhibitors, and the Internet industry. *VNU* is a global information and media company with leading market positions and recognized brands in marketing information (*ACNielsen*), media measurement and information (*Nielsen Media Research*) and business information (*Billboard*, *The Hollywood Reporter*, *Computing*, and *Intermediair*). *VNU* is active in more than one hundred countries, with headquarters in Haarlem, the Netherlands, and New York, USA.

978-0-595-41851-0
0-595-41851-1

Printed in the United States
87527LV00002B/175-999/A